FREEWEIGHT TRAINING ANATOMY

An Illustrated Guide to the Muscles Used While Exercising with Dumbbells, Barbells, Kettlebells and More

RYAN GEORGE

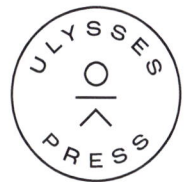

Text copyright © 2016 Ryan George. Design and concept © 2016 Ulysses Press and its licensors. Photographs copyright © 2016 Rapt Productions except as noted below. All rights reserved. Any unauthorized duplication in whole or in part or dissemination of this edition by any means (including but not limited to photocopying, electronic devices, digital versions, and the Internet) will be prosecuted to the fullest extent of the law.

Published in the United States by
Ulysses Press
PO Box 3440
Berkeley, CA 94703
www.ulyssespress.com

ISBN13: 978-1-61243-498-8
Library of Congress Control Number: 2015944218

Printed in the United States
10 9 8 7 6 5 4 3 2 1

Acquisitions editor: Keith Riegert
Managing editor: Claire Chun
Editor: Lily Chou
Proofreader: Lauren Harrison
Interior design: Jake Flaherty
Cover photographs: man © Jasminko Ibrakovic/shutterstock.com; anatomy © TsuneoMP/shutterstock.com
Interior illustrations: © Linda Bucklin/shutterstock.com page 2; © Clip Area/shutterstock.com page 103; © Design 36/shutterstock.com pages 22–27, 36–39, 55, 56 (right), 60, 61, 63, 64, 75–77, 90, 91, 99 (left),102, 107 (left), 108–11, 112, 113 (left), 114; © Digital Storm/shutterstock.com pages 69–72, 95, 96, 99; © DM7/shutterstock.com pages 52–54, 57, 58 (left), 65, 67, 93, 104 (left); © Sebastian Kaulitzki pages 57, 58 (right), 66, 73 (left); © TsuneoMP/shutterstock.com pages 13–20, 29–31, 33–35, 41–43, 45–49, 56 (left), 62, 73 (right), 79, 80, 86–88, 98, 101 (right), 104 (right), 106, 107 (right), 113 (right); © Vitstudio/shutterstock.com pages 82–84; © York Berlin page 101 (left)
Models: Ryan George, Bryan Johnson, Ashley Mitchell
Makeup: Sabrina Foster/SabrinaFosterMakeup.com

Please Note: This book has been written and published strictly for informational purposes, and in no way should be used as a substitute for consultation with health care professionals. You should not consider educational material herein to be the practice of medicine or to replace consultation with a physician or other medical practitioner. The author and publisher are providing you with information in this work so that you can have the knowledge and can choose, at your own risk, to act on that knowledge. The author and publisher also urge all readers to be aware of their health status and to consult health care professionals before beginning any health program.

CONTENTS

PART 1: OVERVIEW — iv
- INTRODUCTION — 1
- FITNESS ESSENTIALS — 3
- USING THIS BOOK — 8

PART 2: EXERCISES — 11
- PECTORALS (CHEST) — 12
- LATISSIMUS DORSI — 21
- UPPER BACK MUSCLES — 28
- DELTOIDS (SHOULDERS) — 32
- BICEPS — 40
- TRICEPS — 44
- TRUNK MUSCLES — 50
- QUADRICEPS — 68
- HAMSTRINGS — 74
- CALF MUSCLES — 78
- GLUTEAL MUSCLES — 81
- OTHER MUSCLES — 85
- FULL-BODY MOVEMENTS — 97

PART 3: THE PROGRAMS — 115
- GETTING STARTED — 116
- PROGRAMMING FOR YOUR GOALS — 123
- EXERCISE PROGRAMS — 126

INDEX — 136
ACKNOWLEDGMENTS — 140
ABOUT THE AUTHOR — 140

PART 1
OVERVIEW

INTRODUCTION

The human body is a remarkably dynamic machine that's capable of producing an incalculable variety of movements. These movements are an essential aspect of how we interact with the world around us. At its core, human movement consists of using our skeletal muscles to manipulate our bones. Maximizing the efficiency as well as the efficacy of movement is important for every single person.

Exercise is the method by which we develop and enhance movement. Obviously, enhancing movement isn't the only reason we exercise; in fact, many people wouldn't consider it the primary or secondary reason, either. We exercise to build muscle mass, lose weight, increase athletic performance, fight off disease, and many other reasons. The one common thread, no matter what the goal, is that exercise is going to involve movement.

There's a reason why I place so much emphasis on movement in exercise. Understanding movements and the muscles that produce them can enhance or severely diminish the effectiveness of an exercise program. When performing even the simplest of movements, it's not simply about an individual muscle or even a "muscle group" working. More often than not, entire movement systems composed of groups of muscles are working synergistically to produce movements. This means that it's important to have a working knowledge of not only what muscles are working when exercising, but also the various roles they play in producing movements. A subtle change in a movement can completely change which muscles and movement systems are involved, so any movements produced during an exercise session should be deliberate and well thought out. Not possessing a working knowledge of the muscles involved in specific movements can, at a minimum, slow development, and, at worst, lead to injury.

The purpose of this book is to give you a variety of exercises using a diverse set of modalities. The exercise descriptions are accompanied by beautiful illustrations to show the specific muscles being used as well as the roles that they play in movement. This knowledge will help you to better design, implement, and follow an exercise program.

In my 15 years in the fitness industry, I've identified guesswork as a very common theme. More often than not, people have very little structure in their exercise program. A combination of the overwhelming amounts of information (and misinformation), conflicting theories, and the new trend of the month often result in confusion. This leads to guesswork and, often, stunted exercise programs.

One of the goals of this book is to simplify exercise. It's not about reinventing the wheel or promoting a brand-new gimmick or fad, but rather giving you the meat and potatoes in a way that's easy to understand. This book consists of the concepts and ideas that I believe to be the most important and instrumental to a successful exercise program. The primary focus is on how to manipulate the muscles of the body in order to perform movements that will in turn help to develop and strengthen those muscles. This information is presented in a way that's concise and easy to digest. In addition to the exercises and illustrations, this book also contains what I believe to be the most important and essential fitness concepts, as well as guidance on designing specific exercise programs for all levels and goals.

Your Body at Work

Skeletal muscles serve a variety of functions. They provide the structure and framework for our bodies. They're used to move bone and allow us to interact with the world. Proper muscular function is important for normal everyday activities as well as athletic performance. Skeletal muscle is also important to many people because of its aesthetic component. We engage in weight training as a way to strengthen, build, and develop skeletal muscle. We can see examples throughout society of well-developed skeletal muscle representing an ideal aspect of the human form.

There are over 200 bones in the human body, and they come in a variety of shapes, sizes, and compositions. Bones serve several different functions but, for the purposes of this book, we'll focus on movement. Together, bones form the skeleton and can be used as a series of levers used to facilitate movement. A joint is an area in which two or more bones meet, allowing for movement. Some joints, like the elbow, move in one direction, while other joints, like the hip, move in more than one direction or have free range to move. Most of the joints throughout the body are acted on by more than one muscle. Understanding the specific movements that a contracted muscle should produce is key to exercise as it allows you to target specific individual muscles and muscle groups.

There are well over 600 skeletal muscles in the human body. Each muscle is individually attached to bones throughout the body. When a muscle contracts, it works to help move a joint in a specific direction. Some muscles, like the hamstrings, act on multiple joints while others, like the soleus, act on only one joint. Groups of individual muscles tend to work together to produce movement. When we refer to muscles, like the quadriceps or the pectorals, we're often referring to a group of muscles that work together. The exercise chapters in this book are separated based on muscle group, and each chapter will break down the individual muscles involved and their role in movement.

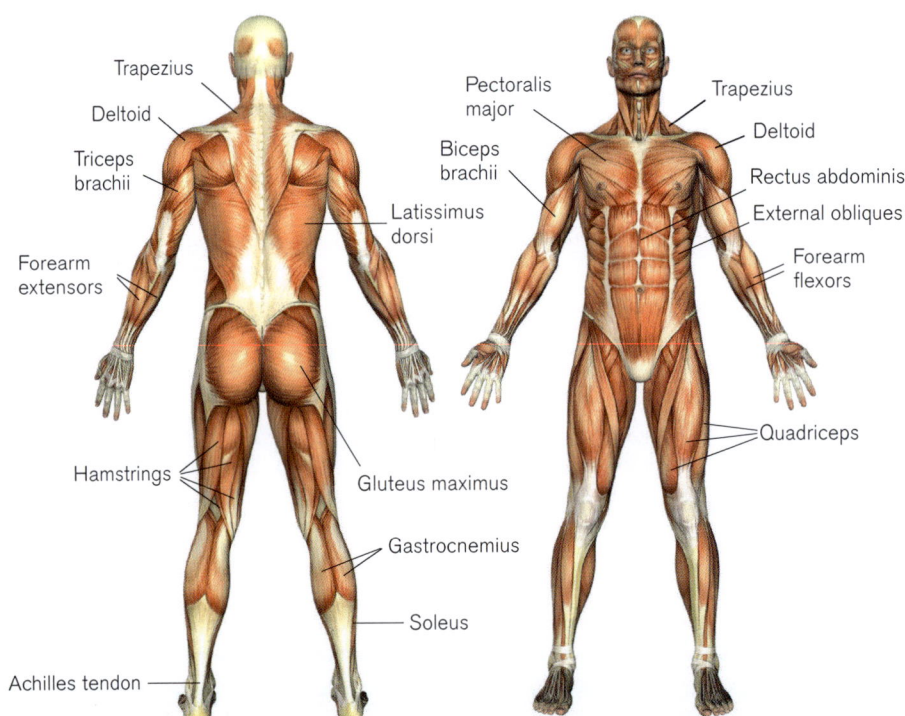

FITNESS ESSENTIALS

In order to eliminate the guesswork that's common in fitness programming, it's necessary to understand a few fitness concepts. This chapter contains what I consider to be the most important concepts that any fitness enthusiast should understand. While following an exercise program doesn't require you to be an expert on fitness, it's necessary to have a basic understanding of exercise science.

Resistance Training

Commonly referred to as strength training or weight training, resistance training refers to exercise in which a person uses some form of muscle contraction to act against an external resistance. The external resistance can vary from a free weight to a machine, or even one's own bodyweight. Resistance training has many benefits. It's commonly used as a way to develop muscular strength, endurance, and size. Resistance training has many other benefits, such as increased bone density, improved mobility, increased metabolic rate, and improved body composition. Almost all of the exercises in this book fall into this category. The exercises and programs in this book will also focus on the muscle-building aspect of resistance training as all of the other benefits will develop as ancillary results if the focus is on muscle building.

Hypertrophy

In the context of resistance training, hypertrophy refers to the enlargement of the muscle tissue. Hypertrophy is a common result of resistance training. To put it simply, when we engage in resistance training, we create microtears in the muscle tissue. The body then reacts to this by repairing tissue larger and stronger in order to better handle the resistance in the future. If you're interested in increasing muscular size, resistance training is the most effective mode to achieve that goal.

Types of Movement

Muscle flexion: The bending of a joint so that the angle decreases. Beginning with a straight arm and bending at the elbow is an example of muscle flexion.

Muscle extension: The straightening of a joint so that the angle increases. Beginning with a bent elbow and straightening the arm is an example of muscle extension.

Hyperextension: Increasing the angle of a joint beyond its normal function.

Abduction: The movement of one segment of the body away from the midline of the body. Lifting the arm to the side is one example of abduction.

Adduction: The movement of one segment of the body toward the midline of the body. Beginning with an arm out to the side and lowering it is an example of adduction.

Rotation: The turning of a segment of the body around an axis. Turning the head to the side is an example of rotation.

Internal rotation: Rotation away from the midline of the body.

External rotation: Rotation toward the midline of the body.

Eversion: Turning a segment of the body outward. Turning the sole of the foot outward is an example.

Inversion: Turning a segment of the body inward. Turning the sole of the foot inward is an example.

Range of Motion

Range of motion (ROM) is the full movement potential of a joint. This is typically measured from full flexion to full extension. Optimal ROM will vary from person to person and may be altered due to injury. ROM plays an important role in exercise and most movements should be performed throughout the optimal ROM.

Types of Exercise

Isolation exercises: These exercises tend to focus on the movement of one joint. This is done as a way to increase the focus on one muscle while eliminating any unwanted assistance to the movement. A dumbbell hammer curl (see page 42) is an example of an isolation exercise since the elbow joint is the only joint moving.

Compound exercises: These exercises are movements that involve the use of two or more joints. These movements use one or more muscle groups at a time, allowing for significantly more resistance and variety. A squat is an example of a compound exercise since the hip, knee, and ankle joints all work simultaneously.

Functional exercises: Designed to mimic movements that people encounter in everyday life, these exercises are particularly useful for athletes, older populations, and people recovering from injuries. Appropriate functional exercises will vary greatly based on the individual.

Types of Muscle Contraction

Concentric: Concentric contraction occurs when the muscle fibers shorten as muscular tension is produced.

Exercise application: During traditional resistance training, the prime and assistant movers work together to produce a concentric contraction to overcome an external resistance.

Eccentric: Eccentric contraction occurs when the muscle fibers lengthen as muscular tension is produced.

Exercise application: During traditional resistance training, the prime and assistant movers work together to produce an eccentric contraction in order to decelerate or control an external resistance.

Isometric: Isometric contraction occurs when muscle fibers remain static while producing tension.

Exercise application: During traditional resistance training, the prime and assistant movers will produce an isometric contraction momentarily during the transition from concentric to eccentric or eccentric to concentric. Stabilizer muscles also produce an isometric contraction in order to maintain stability throughout a movement.

Breathing

It's important to focus on your breathing during resistance training. It's generally best to exhale during the concentric portion of the movement and inhale during the eccentric portion of the movement. During isometric exercises, simply maintain consistent breathing thought the exercise.

The easiest way to determine when to exhale or inhale is to remember to exhale when you're exerting force and to inhale when you're controlling the weight down. Since all of the exercises in this book use free weights or bodyweight, it's even easier to figure this out. We're exerting force whenever we move an object up, against gravity. This means that whenever we're moving ourselves or an object up, we should exhale; whenever we're moving ourselves or an object down, we should control the resistance down and inhale.

Components of a Movement

When we perform any movement, our muscles work together in a variety of ways to produce that movement. From typing on a keyboard to performing a back flip, every movement requires precise and specific coordination of muscles throughout the body to be successful. When exercising, knowing the different roles that the muscles play will go a long way toward maximizing the training effect of any exercise.

Prime mover: While most movements involve the use of multiple muscles, one muscle typically produces a majority of the force against the external resistance. In traditional resistance training, the prime mover is the muscle producing the concentric action. This muscle is also referred to as the agonist. When performing a push-up, the pectorals (chest muscles) would be considered the prime mover.

Assistant movers: These provide additional force and assist the prime movers in producing a movement. During some movements, an assistant mover may switch over to being the prime mover at some point in the ROM. During a push-up, the triceps work as assistant movers but are the prime mover at the top of the ROM.

Antagonist: This is the muscle that produces the opposing force to a given movement. While the agonist produces the concentric action, the antagonist produces the eccentric action. Agonist and antagonist muscles often work in pairs. The eccentric action of the antagonist muscles are important because they help to maintain control and stability during movements. During a push-up, the posterior deltoids, rhomboids, trapezius, and biceps all contract eccentrically to oppose the prime and assistant movers.

Stabilizer: Incredibly important to movement, stabilizer muscles essentially hold bones and parts of the body in place while other muscles work to produce the movement. In order to maintain stability, stabilizer muscles contract isometrically. During a push-up, all of the core muscles contract isometrically in order to maintain stability of the spine during the movement.

Fitness Principles and Concept

The following are essential principles that should be followed as closely as possible. Whether you're a novice or a professional, adhering to these principles will make success far more likely.

Specificity: The specificity principle says that your body will adapt specifically to the kind of exercise that you participate in. The more specific the goal or skill, the more specific the training needs to be. A marathon runner, for example, needs a high level of aerobic endurance. Activities like long-distance running, cycling, and swimming are all beneficial since they help develop aerobic endurance. Heavyweight training, on the other hand, wouldn't translate as well because it doesn't focus on aerobic endurance.

Consistency: For most people, consistency is the single most important factor in determining the success of a fitness program. While the body is great at adapting to stress, the opposite is also true. Commonly referred to as the "use it or lose it" principle, the body will regress if you don't provide it with sufficient stress in the form of exercise. All it takes is 10 days for muscles to atrophy and to lose a significant amount of your aerobic capacity.

Consistency is also important because, ideally, exercise should be a part of your lifestyle. Most people aren't passionate about exercise so it's important to find a routine that's manageable but consistent in order to make it a regular thing. It's easy to make excuses and skip training. I've witnessed time and time again how an inconsistent regimen can quickly turn into an extended absence from exercise. Over time, a consistent program should ingrain itself into your life.

Efficiency: When it comes to improving your fitness, in most situations you should emphasize quality over quantity. It's important to maximize your time exercising. Using programs like high-intensity interval training (HIIT), you can get more work done in a 20-minute workout than you can in an hour of traditional training. This helps to eliminate time as an obstacle. The key is to work as hard as you can, with minimal rest over a short period of time.

Progression: As I mentioned earlier, we benefit from exercise because our body has to adapt to new stress and stimuli. If we don't introduce new stress, the body has no need to adapt and may therefore regress. This is often the cause of the dreaded plateau. The principle of progression, or progressive overload, says that we must constantly and consistently push ourselves beyond what our bodies are used to in order to progress.

Rest and recovery: Rest and recovery are very commonly overlooked when developing an exercise program. When you exercise, you place stress on the body, breaking it down a little. While resting, your body adapts by rebuilding itself stronger. If you don't allow yourself time to recover, exercise starts to follow the law of diminishing returns. Too little rest can lead to overtraining, which can then lead to physical regression and injuries. Optimal rest time varies based on your current fitness level as well as the activity, but most people should have at least two rest days per week.

Other Important Fitness Concepts

Plateau: Sometimes we reach a point in an exercise program where, no matter how much we try, we can't seem to make any progress. This is often referred to as a plateau and is usually a sign that we need to change things up.

Periodization: Periodization is a method of changing a fitness program in set intervals. Usually, each cycle has its own set of specific goals. This is a great way to fight a plateau as you never stick with one training method for too long. To give an example, if my ultimate goal is to both add 10 pounds of muscle and lose 10 pounds of fat, a periodized program would be the most efficient. The two goals conflict quite a bit and it would be difficult to both add 10 pounds of muscle and lose 10 pounds of fat using the same program. With a periodized program, I'd spend 8 to 12 weeks focused only on muscle building. Once I've added the 10 pounds of muscle, I'd focus on a fat-loss program.

Plyometrics: This is a form of training that utilizes what's called the stretch shortening cycle. In the strictest sense, it refers to exercises done so explosively that they rely on the body's production of elastic energy. Oftentimes, power exercises like squat jumps and burpees get mistakenly called plyometrics. While they're power exercises, they don't quite fit into the true definition.

Overtraining: Overtraining happens when a person gets too much exercise, too little rest, or a combination of the two. When designing an exercise program, it's important to consider your current condition. While progression is important, it should be gradual. Signs of overtraining include increased injuries, constant soreness, unusual fatigue, and irritability.

USING THIS BOOK

Part 2 of this book contains the list of illustrated exercises. The exercises cover muscles throughout the body and are categorized by muscle group. Each exercise description contains full-color illustrations, detailed instruction, and an explanation of how the muscles are involved in the movement. The emphasis on how the muscles contribute to specific movements are useful to fitness enthusiasts of all levels, from novice exercisers to fitness professionals.

Part 3 of this book consists of some very useful information on designing an exercise program to meet your goals. Pre-set exercise programs are included, as well as information on cardio and flexibility. The pre-set exercise programs are organized by fitness goals and are highly recommended for beginner and novice readers. While these programs are effective for all levels, those with more of a DIY approach to exercise can find detailed information on designing an exercise program.

Understanding the Exercise Description

Name: Name of the exercise

Equipment: The equipment that's necessary for the exercise

Prime movers: These are the muscles that are primarily responsible for the movement. In some cases, individual muscles will be referenced and, in others, entire muscle groups will be referenced.

Assistant movers: The muscles that assist in the movement

Stabilizers: These are the muscles that stabilize the body while producing the movement. In some instances, the stabilizing muscles are the muscles that you should be focusing on; in those instances the muscles will be noted.

Prerequisite exercises: The exercises that you should be familiar with before attempting

1. Each number represents the different steps in the exercise.

Notes: Important points about positioning and movement to be mindful of

Progressions: Ways to make the exercise more challenging

Regressions: Ways to modify the exercise if it's too difficult

Equipment

Most of the exercises in this book utilize some form of freeweight training, which means exercising with a weighted object that's not controlled by any external forces. Exercising with free weights requires you to be 100 percent responsible for producing a desired movement. The benefit is that your entire body has to function as a unit to produce a movement as opposed to working with a machine that will help to guide your body through a movement.

Bodyweight: Bodyweight exercises use your own bodyweight as resistance.

Barbell: A free weight in the form of a bar that's meant to be used by both arms together. They may vary in length and can be loaded with weight.

Dumbbell: A small version of a barbell meant to be handled in one hand.

Kettlebell: A weight that's typically made of cast iron in the shape of a round bell with a handle on the top. The shape and handle make them more useful for a variety of functional and momentum-based movements.

Physioball: An inflatable ball that varies from 35 to 90cm in diameter, its unstable surface makes it useful for a variety of things. It can be used in combination with other equipment or as a way to make a traditional bodyweight exercise more difficult.

Sandbag: Typically designed with handles to increase functionality, these are typically bags weighed down with sand, rocks, water, or other material. They're great for functional training.

Medicine ball: A weighted ball ranging from 2 pounds to 30 pounds that can be made of a variety of materials. It's great for functional training.

Positioning

While there may be some differences based on the specific requirements for the exercise, every exercise begins in one of the following positions.

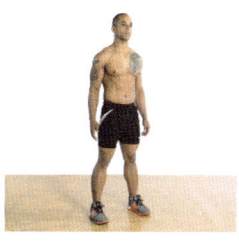

Standing Upright

Feet: Hip- to shoulder-width apart with the toes pointing straight ahead
Knees: Slightly bent
Lower Back: Slight arch
Upper Back: Shoulder blades together
Head: Ears in line with the shoulders

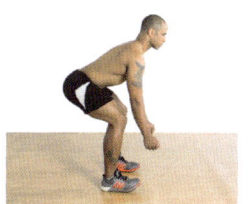

Standing, Bent Over

Feet: Hip- to shoulder-width apart with the toes pointing straight ahead
Knees: Bent
Torso: Bent over as close to parallel to the floor while maintaining a straight back
Upper Back: Shoulder blades together

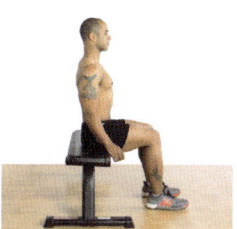

Seated

Feet: Hip- to shoulder-width apart with the toes pointing straight ahead
Knees: Bent 90 degrees
Hips: Thighs bent 90 degrees at the hip
Lower Back: Slight arch
Upper Back: Shoulder blades together
Head: Ears in line with the shoulders

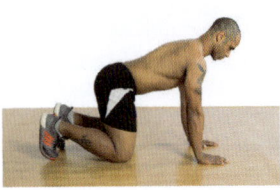

Quadruped Position

Feet: Hip- to shoulder-width apart
Knees: Bent 90 degrees and touching the floor
Hips: Bent 90 degrees
Lower Back: Sight arch
Upper Back: Shoulder blades together
Arms: Extended with the hands directly under the shoulders and touching the floor
Head: In line with the feet, knees, hips, and shoulders

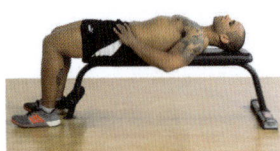

Lying Supine

Feet: Shoulder-width apart and flat on the floor or bench, pointing straight ahead
Lower Back: Slight arch
Upper Back: Shoulder blades together
Head: Back of the head on the floor or bench

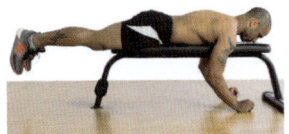

Lying Prone

Feet: Hip- to shoulder-width apart
Knees: Slightly bent
Hips: In line with the feet and knees
Lower Back: Sight arch
Upper Back: Shoulder blades together
Head: In line with the feet, knees, hips, and shoulders

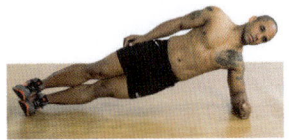

Side Lying

Feet, knees, hips, spine, and head should be in line

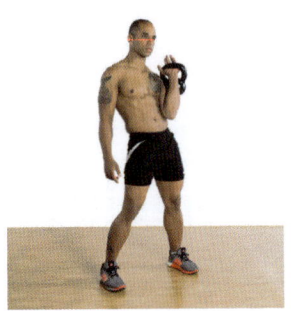

Catch Position (with a Kettlebell)

Feet: Hip- to shoulder-width apart with toes pointing straight ahead
Knees: Bent slightly
Lower Back: Slight arch and leaning back slightly
Upper Back: Shoulder blades together
Arms: Holding a kettlebell at chest level, with palms in a neutral position and arms resting on the trunk
Head: Ears in line with the shoulders

PART 2
EXERCISES

PECTORALS (CHEST)

The pectorals are the muscles located on the chest. The group consists of two muscles, the pectoralis major and the pectoralis minor.

Muscles & Actions

Pectoralis major: Composed of two heads, the pectoralis major horizontally abducts and internally rotates the humerus, the largest bone in the arm. The clavicular head is located at the upper portion of the chest near the shoulders; the sternal head is located at the lower portion of the pectoralis major. In addition to the above movements, the clavicular head assists in horizontal abduction when the arm is at 110 degrees. The sternal head assists with downward extension of an elevated arm.

Pectoralis minor: The pectoralis minor is located underneath the pectoralis major and draws the scapula downward and forward.

Training Tips

- It's important to maintain stability in the shoulder when performing chest exercises as rotator cuff injuries can occur with improper form.

- Exercises performed at an incline are effective in developing the upper, clavicular portion of the pectoralis.

- While pressing exercises like the Bench Press (page 14) and Dumbbell Press (page 15) should be staples in any strength-training routine, they rely heavily on the triceps and shoulders as assistant movers. Exercises that focus exclusively on horizontal abduction, like the Dumbbell Fly (page 16), can be effective because they isolate the muscles and rely minimally on the assistant movers.

PECTORALS (CHEST)

Push-Up

EQUIPMENT: None

PRIME MOVERS: Pectoralis major, triceps

ASSISTANT MOVERS: Anterior deltoids, pectoralis minor

STABILIZERS: Rotator cuff muscles, serratus anterior, oblique muscles, rectus abdominis, erector spinae

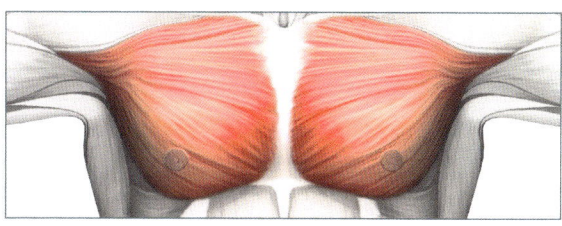
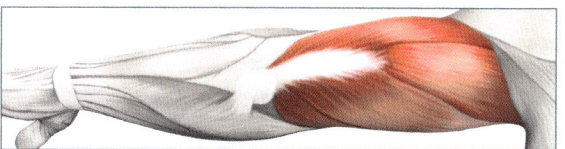

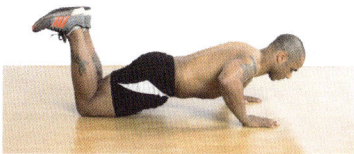

REGRESSION

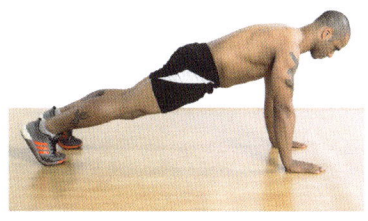
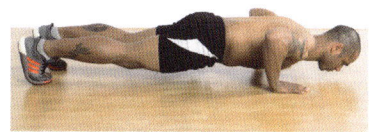

1. Facing the floor, place your hands on the floor directly under your shoulders and extend your legs behind you. Your hands and toes should be the only points of contact on the floor and your body should be in a neutral position, with a straight line from your shoulders, through your back, and to your ankles.

2. Maintaining a straight back throughout the movement, bend your elbows out to the sides and lower yourself to the floor; be careful not to overarch your lower back. At the middle of the movement, your chest should be as low to the floor as you can comfortably get with your elbows out to the side.

Return to the starting position.

- Place your knees on the floor and perform the push-up.
- Shorten the ROM to one half or three fourths.

NOTES

- Maintain a neutral neck position throughout.
- A wider hand position will reduce assistance coming from the triceps and anterior deltoids, placing more of a focus on the pectoralis, while a narrower hand position will increase assistance coming from the triceps.

Bench Press

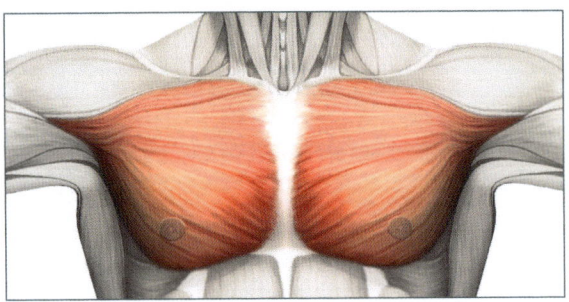

EQUIPMENT: Barbell

PRIME MOVER: Pectoralis major

ASSISTANT MOVERS: Triceps, anterior deltoids

STABILIZERS: Rotator cuff muscles, core muscles, forearm muscles

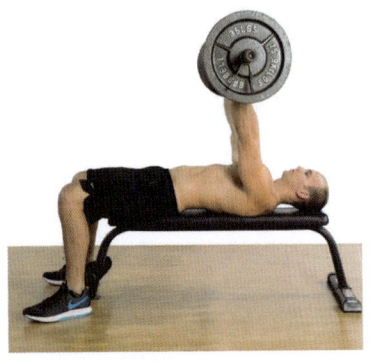

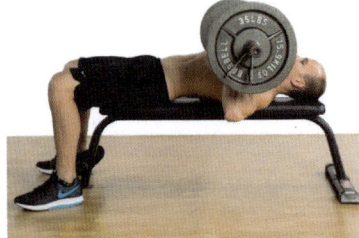

1. Lie face-up on a bench with your chest underneath the bar. Grip the bar with your hands slightly wider than shoulder-width apart.

2. Bend your elbows out to the sides and lower the bar toward your chest until it's 3 to 6 inches above your chest.

Press the bar back up to the starting position.

NOTES

- Lowering the bar to the point of touching your chest can be potentially harmful to your shoulders and unnecessary for developing your chest.
- Make sure to keep your abdominals braced and don't overarch your lower back.
- Changing your hand position will alter how your muscles work. A wider grip will focus more on the pectoralis major but you'll receive less assistance from the triceps and shoulders. A narrower grip will place more emphasis on the triceps and less on the pectoralis major.

PECTORALS (CHEST)

Dumbbell Press

EQUIPMENT: Dumbbells

PRIME MOVER: Pectoralis major

ASSISTANT MOVERS: Triceps, anterior deltoids

STABILIZERS: Core muscles, rotator cuff muscles, forearm muscles

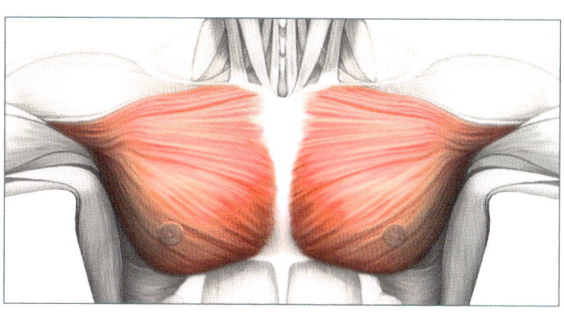

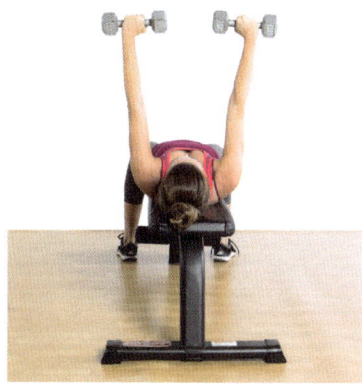

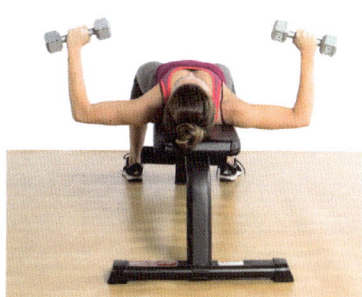

PROGRESSION

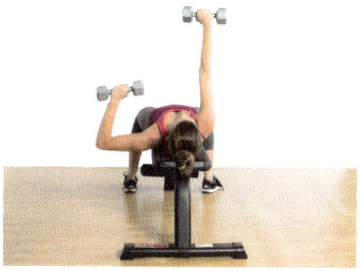

- Begin with both arms in the starting position and press with one arm at a time.

REGRESSION

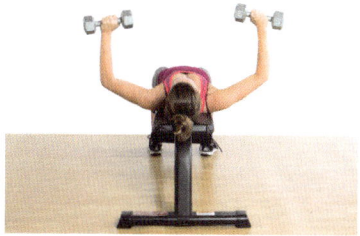

- Shorten the ROM to one half or three fourths.

1. Lie face-up on a bench with your feet touching the floor. Hold a dumbbell in each hand with your arms fully extended over your shoulders.

2. Bend your elbows and horizontally abduct your shoulders, lowering the dumbbells to the sides. Movement at the elbows and shoulders should be even, creating an arc that's not too wide or too narrow. At the middle of the movement, your upper arms should be slightly below parallel, with your elbows bent approximately 90 degrees.

Squeeze your chest and drive through your palms, tracing the arc back up to the starting position.

NOTES

- Press at an incline to assist in developing the clavicular portion of the pectoralis major.

- Press at a decline to assist in developing the sternal portion of the pectoralis major.

Dumbbell Fly

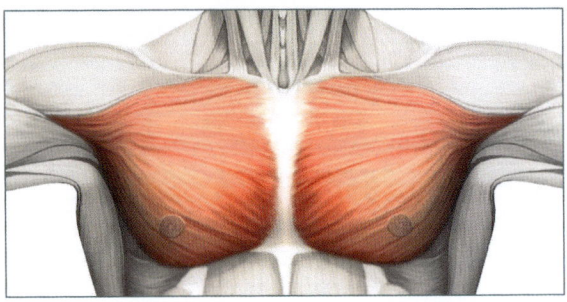

EQUIPMENT: **Dumbbells**
PRIME MOVER: **Pectoralis major**
ASSISTANT MOVERS: **Anterior deltoids**
STABILIZERS: **Biceps, triceps, forearm muscles**

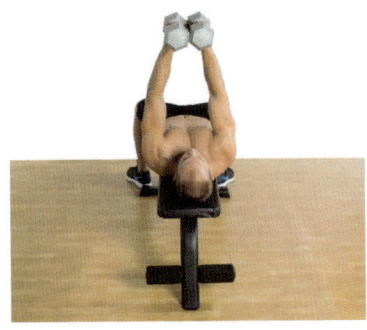

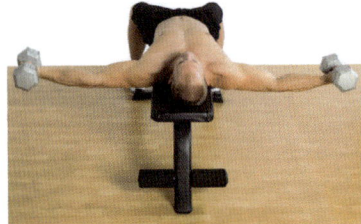

1. Lie face-up on a bench. Hold a dumbbell in each hand with your arms extended upward with your palms facing each other. Your elbows should be slightly bent.

2. Keeping your elbows locked in place but maintaining the same angle as the starting position, lower until your arms are slightly below parallel to the floor.

Horizontally adduct your arms back to the starting position.

> **NOTES**
> - Make sure to maintain stability in your shoulder blades as well as your elbows. All of the movement should be at the shoulders.

PECTORALS (CHEST)

Bench Pullover

EQUIPMENT: Dumbbell

PRIME MOVER: Pectoralis major

ASSISTANT MOVERS: Latissimus dorsi, teres major

STABILIZERS: Biceps, triceps, deltoids, rectus abdominis, forearm muscles

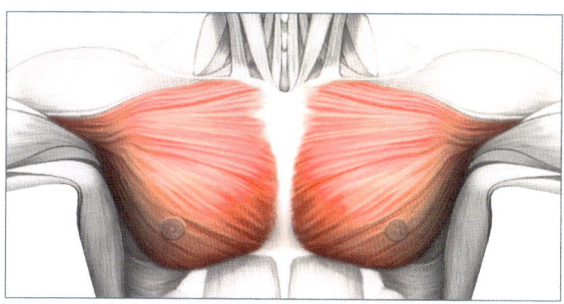

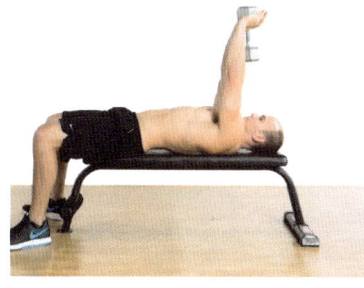

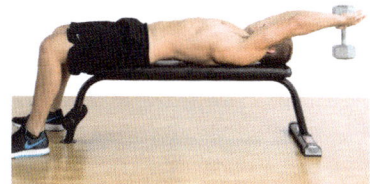

1. Lie face-up on a bench. Hold one dumbbell in between your hands and fully extend your arms upward.

2. Bracing the abdominals to avoid overarching your lower back throughout the movement, lower your arms back toward the floor behind you. The movement should only occur at your shoulders and your elbows should remain stable throughout the movement. At the bottom of the movement, your arms should extend as far as they comfortably can without pain or discomfort in the shoulders or lower back.

Pull the weight back to the starting position, making sure to keep your elbows locked and stable throughout.

NOTES

- This movement places more emphasis on the sternal portion of the pectoralis major.

FREEWEIGHT TRAINING ANATOMY

Kettlebell Press

EQUIPMENT: Kettlebell
PRIME MOVER: Pectoralis major
ASSISTANT MOVERS: Triceps
STABILIZERS: Rotator cuff muscles, core muscles, forearm muscles

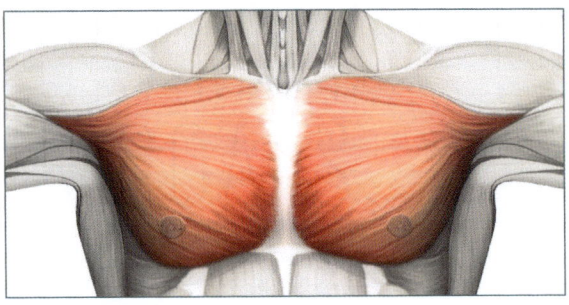

PROGRESSION

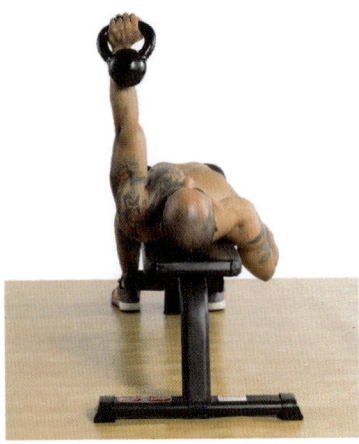

1. Lie face-up on a bench with a kettlebell in one hand. Fully extend that arm with your palm in a neutral position.

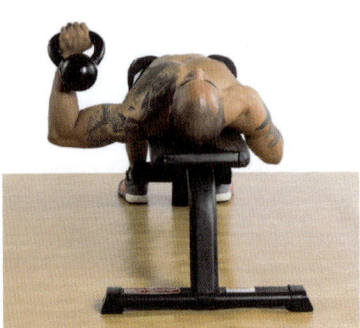

2. Brace your core and lower your arm with your elbow out to the side. At the bottom of the movement, your hand should be in line with your chest.

Press back up to the starting position.

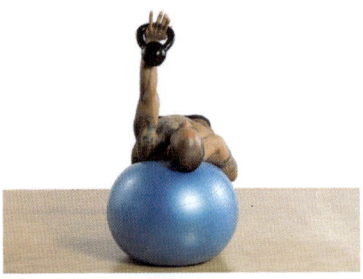

- Do the exercise while lying on a physioball.

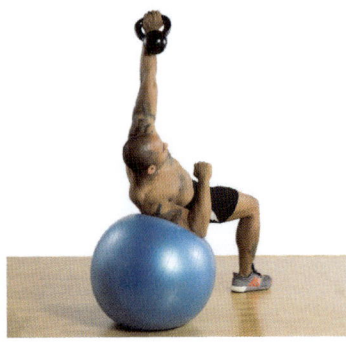

- While still on a physioball, add torso rotation to the top of the movement by lifting the side holding the kettlebell off of the ball.

NOTES
- In addition to the chest, this is a great core workout as you must engage your core in order to stay stable throughout the movement.

PECTORALS (CHEST) 19

Physioball Push-Up

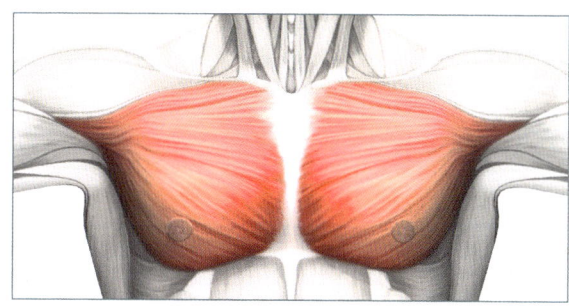

EQUIPMENT: Physioball

PRIME MOVER: Pectoralis major

ASSISTANT MOVERS: Deltoids, triceps

STABILIZERS: Core muscles, quadriceps, hamstrings, gluteal muscles

PREREQUISITE EXERCISE: Push-up (page 13)

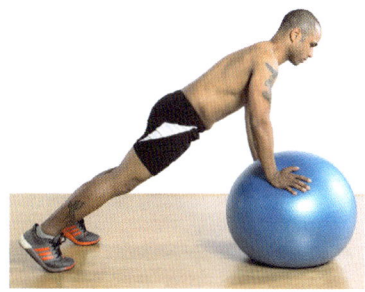 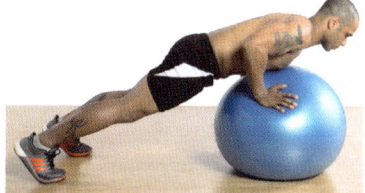

1. Place your hands on a physioball and assume the top of a push-up position.

2. Lower down until your chest lightly touches the physioball.

Press back up through your palms to the starting position.

Explosive Push-Up

EQUIPMENT: None
PRIME MOVER: Pectoralis major
ASSISTANT MOVERS: Triceps, anterior deltoids, quadriceps
STABILIZERS: Core muscles, rotator cuff muscles
PREREQUISITE EXERCISES: Push-up (page 13)

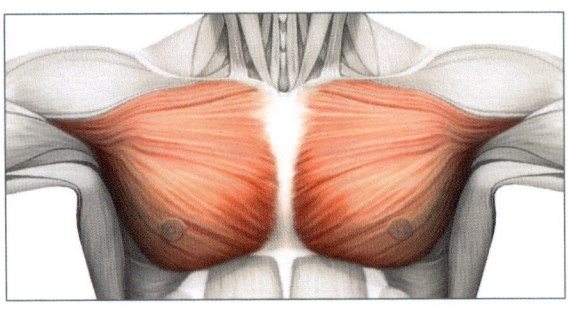

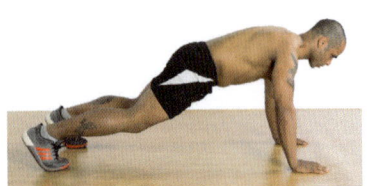

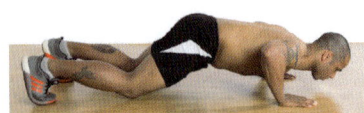

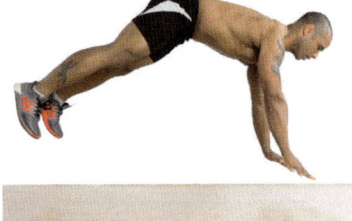

1. Assume the top of a push-up position. Your knees should be slightly bent.

2. Lower yourself to the floor by bending your elbows out to the sides. As you lower yourself, bend your knees a bit more. At the bottom of the movement, your trunk should remain stable and your chest should be 3 to 6 inches off of the floor.

3. In one motion, explosively drive through your palms and extend your legs, lifting your entire body off of the floor. At the top of the movement, your arms should be fully extended toward the floor. You should be as high off of the floor as you can comfortably get.

Absorb the impact of the landing by bending your elbows prior to touching the floor. Upon impact, continue to lower into the next repetition.

REGRESSION

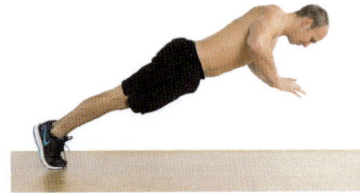

- Keep your feet on the floor.

NOTES

- A soft landing is a crucial part of protecting against injuries.
- As an explosive movement, it's important to perform each repetition as quickly and powerfully as you can.

LATISSIMUS DORSI

The latissimus dorsi (lats) is the largest muscle in the back. A dynamic muscle that's often underutilized in strength training, it's an important muscle that's responsible for a variety of upper-body movements.

Muscles & Actions

The latissimus dorsi is responsible for extension, adduction, internal rotation, and horizontal abduction of the shoulder joint.

Training Tips

- The latissimus dorsi is capable of a wide variety of movements. Any training program should reflect this variety.
- Straight-arm movements like dumbbell pullovers are great for isolating the latissimus dorsi, while multi-joint movements like rows are great for lifting heavier weights.
- Avoid a protracted (shoulders forward) position when performing exercises for the latissimus dorsi.
- It's easy to overuse the biceps when performing certain exercises, so try to focus on pulling from the latissimus dorsi and squeezing the muscle at the top of the movement.

Straight-Arm Dumbbell Extension

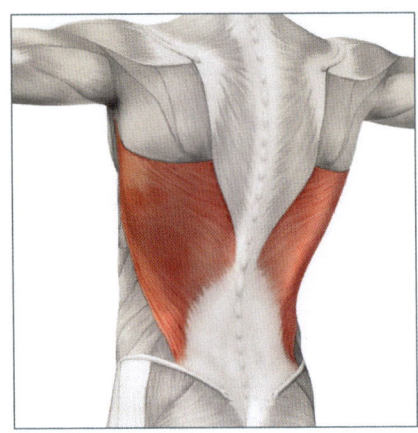

EQUIPMENT: Dumbbell

PRIME MOVER: Latissimus dorsi

ASSISTANT MOVER: Pectoralis major

STABILIZERS: Biceps, triceps, forearm muscles

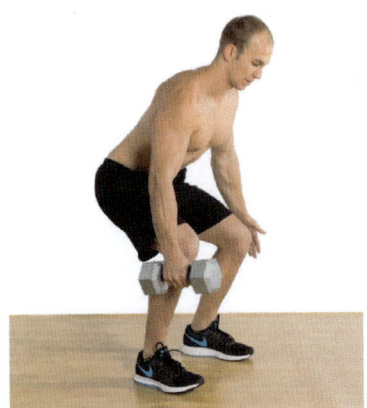

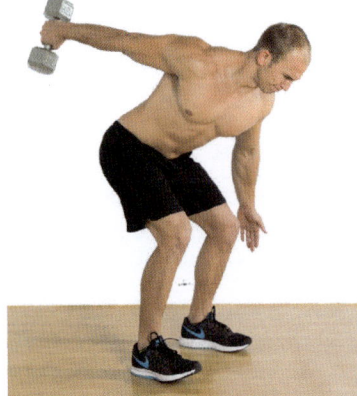

1. Stand in a bent-over position with a dumbbell in one hand and your palms facing each other. Your arms should be fully extended.

2. Moving only at the shoulder, extend the arm holding the dumbbell behind you until it's parallel to the floor.

Lower your arm back to the starting position.

LATISSIMUS DORSI   23

One-Arm Dumbbell Row

EQUIPMENT: Dumbbell

PRIME MOVER: Latissimus dorsi

ASSISTANT MOVERS: Biceps, trapezius, rhomboids

STABILIZERS: Forearm muscles, core muscles

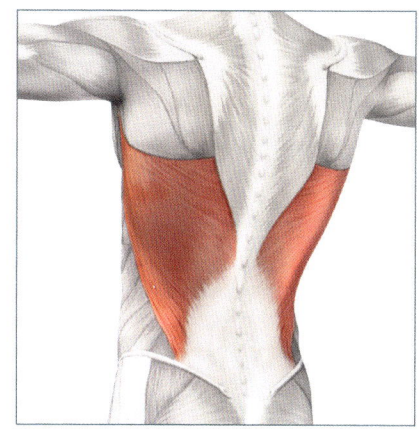

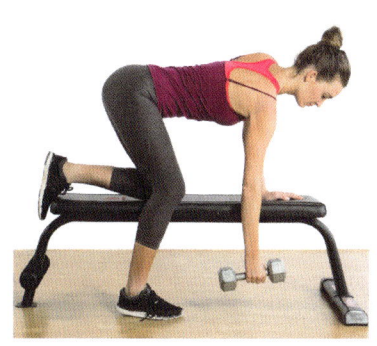
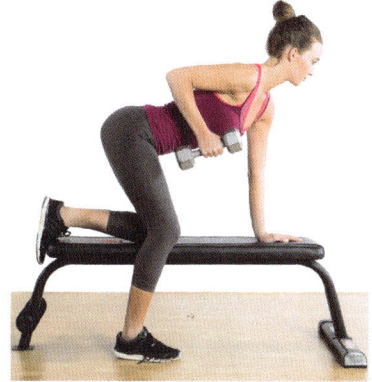

1. Stand in a bent-over position with your left knee and left hand on a bench. Your right foot should be on the floor and your right arm should be holding a dumbbell with your palm in a neutral position. Your back should be straight and your core engaged.

2. While maintaining a stable trunk, squeeze your shoulder blades together and pull the dumbbell up. At the top of the movement, your hand should be in line with your chest and your upper arm close to your torso.

Lower the dumbbell back to the starting position.

NOTES

- Maintain a stable trunk throughout the movement. Don't rotate or shift your weight.

Two-Arm Dumbbell Row

EQUIPMENT: Dumbbells

PRIME MOVER: Latissimus dorsi

ASSISTANT MOVERS: Biceps, trapezius, rhomboids

STABILIZERS: Core muscles, forearm muscles

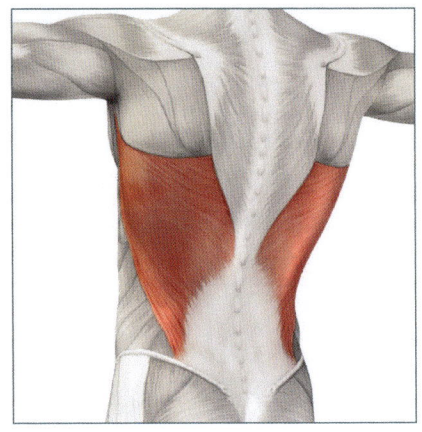

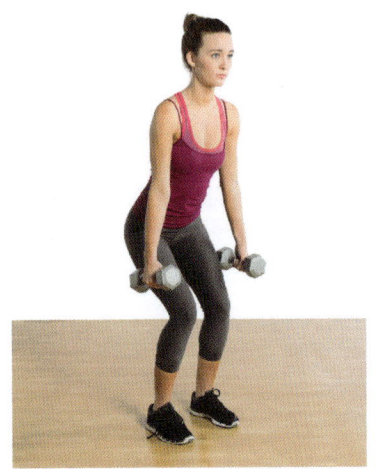

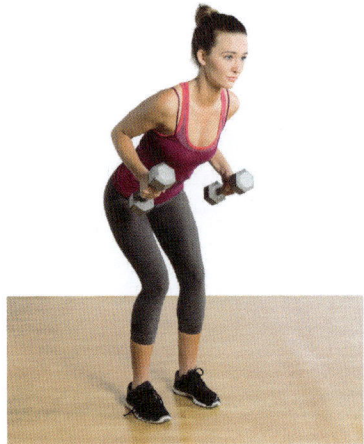

PROGRESSION

- Begin at the midpoint. Use one arm at a time while keeping the other arm static at the top of the movement.

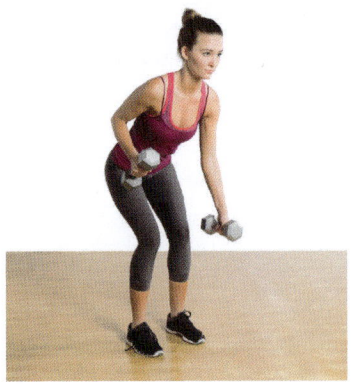

1. Stand in a bent-over position with a dumbbell in each hand and your palms facing each other. Your arms should be fully extended and hanging down toward the floor.

2. Squeeze your shoulder blades together and pull the dumbbells straight up until they're in line with your chest. Keep your elbows close to your torso. Lower the dumbbells back to the starting position. Release your shoulder blades once your arms are fully extended.

LATISSIMUS DORSI 25

Decline Dumbbell Pullover

EQUIPMENT: Dumbbell

PRIME MOVERS: Latissimus dorsi, pectoralis major

ASSISTANT MOVER: Serratus anterior

STABILIZERS: Core muscles, biceps, triceps, forearm muscles

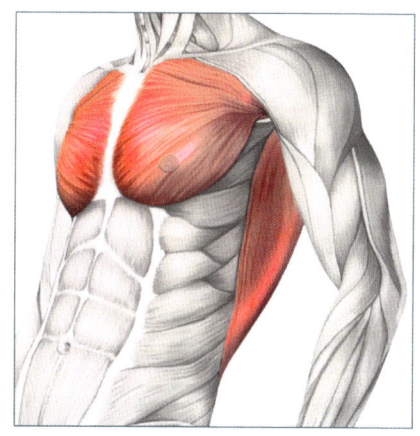

PROGRESSION

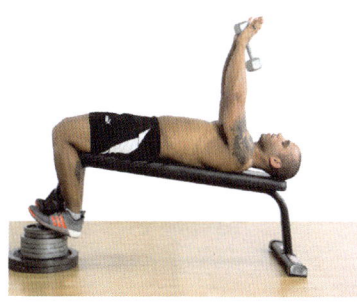

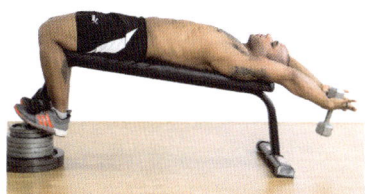

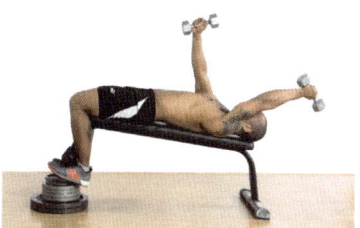

1. Lie face-up on a decline bench with your head on the lower end. Your arms should be holding a dumbbell from one end with your arms fully extended and perpendicular to the floor.

2. Keeping your elbows locked and straight throughout the movement, slowly lower your arms back toward the floor as far as you can comfortably get them. Your elbows should be fully extended and your lower back should not be overarched.

Pull the dumbbell back to the starting position.

- Hold one dumbbell in each hand and alternate arms.

NOTES
- Maintain a stable lower back.

Single-Leg Kettlebell Row

EQUIPMENT: Kettlebell

PRIME MOVER: Latissimus dorsi

ASSISTANT MOVERS: Rhomboids, biceps

STABILIZERS: Core muscles, hamstrings, quadriceps, forearm muscles, calves

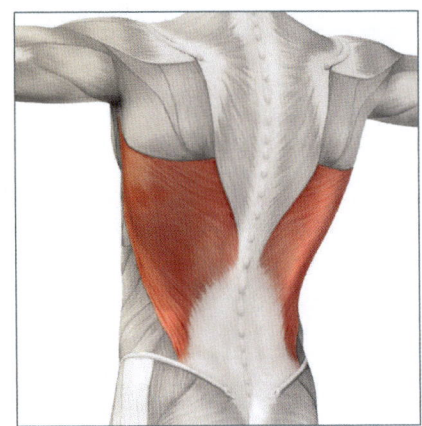

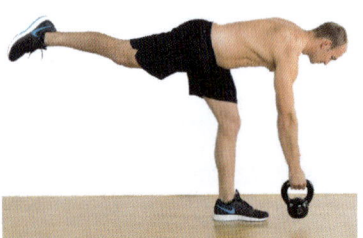

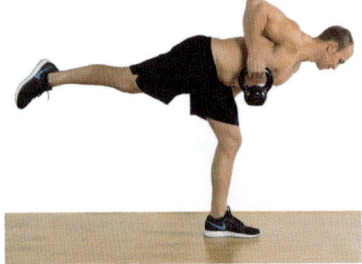

REGRESSION

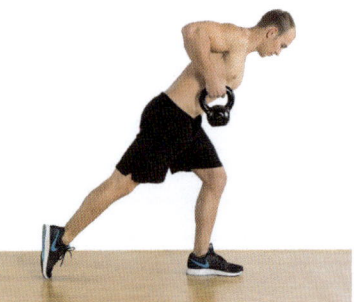

1. Stand on your left leg with your torso parallel to the floor and your right leg fully extended behind you and in line with your torso. Hold a dumbbell in your right hand with your arm fully extended and pointing toward the floor.

2. While maintaining your stability and keeping your arm close to your torso, pull the kettlebell up until it's in line with your chest.

Maintaining your stability, lower the kettlebell back to the starting position.

- If balance is an issue, lower your back foot and lightly touch the floor.

LATISSIMUS DORSI 27

Pull-Up

EQUIPMENT: Pull-up bar

PRIME MOVER: Latissimus dorsi

ASSISTANT MOVERS: Trapezius, biceps, posterior deltoid

STABILIZERS: Forearm muscles

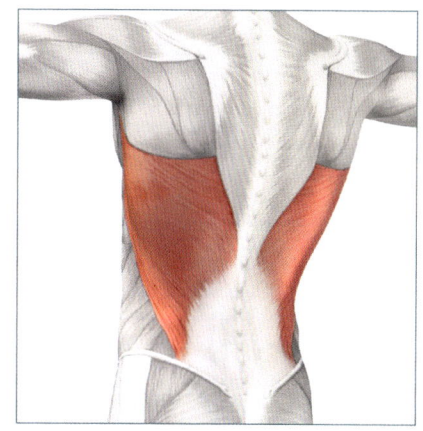

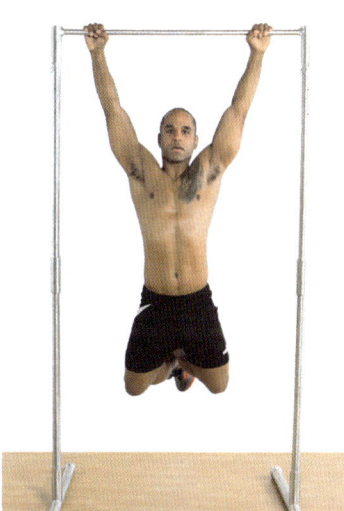

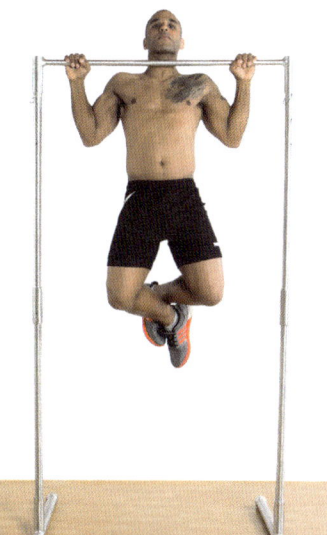

REGRESSION

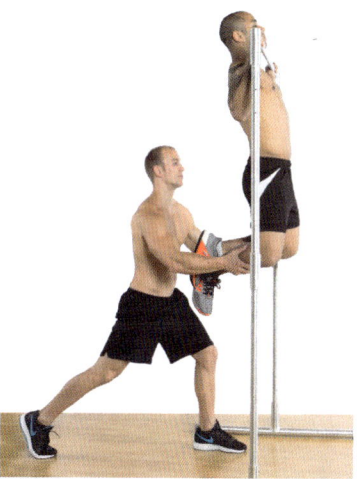

1. Hang on a bar with your arms fully extended and slightly wider than shoulder-width apart.

2. Squeeze your shoulder blades together and pull yourself up toward the bar until your chin is 2 to 3 inches above the bar with your elbows out to the sides.

Keeping your shoulder blades together until your arms are fully extended, lower yourself back down.

- Have a partner assist you. You can do this by hanging with your knees bent behind you and placing your feet in your partner's hands. Your partner can then assist as much as is necessary.

UPPER BACK MUSCLES

The muscles of the upper back are typically responsible for producing horizontal abduction of the humerus, retraction of the shoulder blades, and elevation of the shoulders.

Muscles & Actions

Pectoralis minor: Located underneath the pectoralis major, it draws the scapula downward and forward.

Trapezius: Split into three portions, the upper trapezius is responsible for elevation of the shoulders; the middle trapezius is responsible for scapular retraction; and the lower trapezius is responsible for the depression and retraction of the scapulae.

Rhomboids: Retraction of the scapulae; important for stability of the shoulder girdle.

Posterior Deltoid: Horizontal abduction of the humerus. A part of the deltoid muscle group, the deltoids also work with the upper back muscles.

Training Tips

- When training the upper back, arm position is an important component. Generally, upper back exercises should be performed with your arms abducted; otherwise, the lats will be heavily involved. Take the barbell row, for example. If the arm aren't abducted, the primary mover becomes the latissimus dorsi.

- Avoid elevation of the shoulders when performing upper back movements.

Dumbbell Shrug

EQUIPMENT: Dumbbells

PRIME MOVER: Trapezius (upper portion)

ASSISTANT MOVERS: Rhomboids

STABILIZERS: Biceps, triceps, forearms

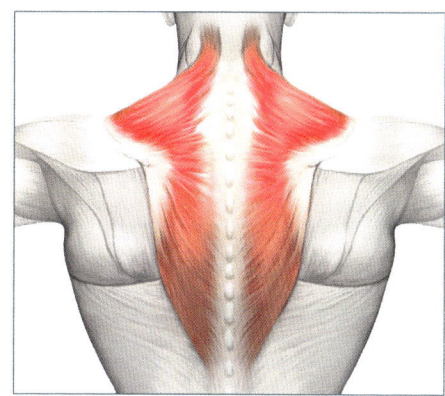

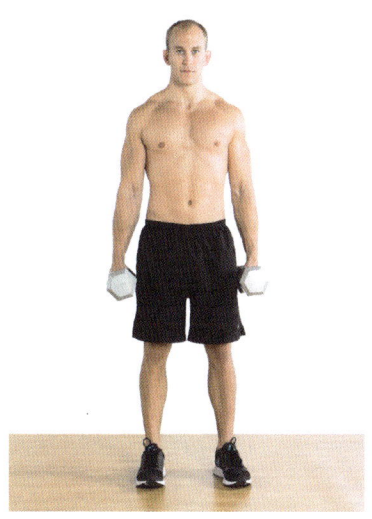

1. Stand upright with a dumbbell in each hand with your arms extended.

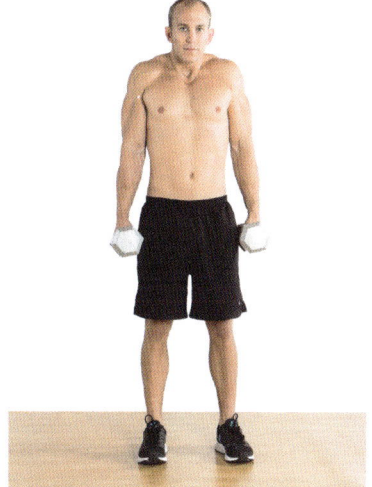

2. Keeping your neck in a neutral position throughout, raise your shoulders to your ears while squeezing your shoulder blades together.

Lower back to the starting position.

Dumbbell Scapular Retraction

EQUIPMENT: Dumbbells

PRIME MOVERS: Rhomboids, trapezius (middle and lower portions)

ASSISTANT MOVER: Teres major

STABILIZERS: Core muscles, forearm muscles

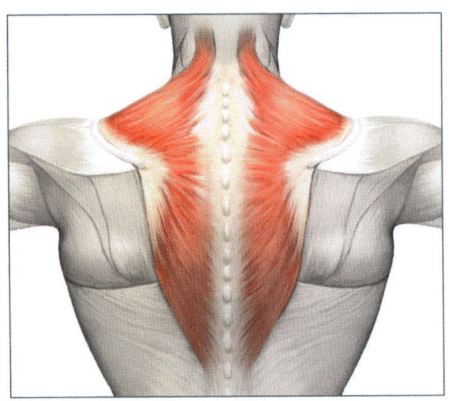

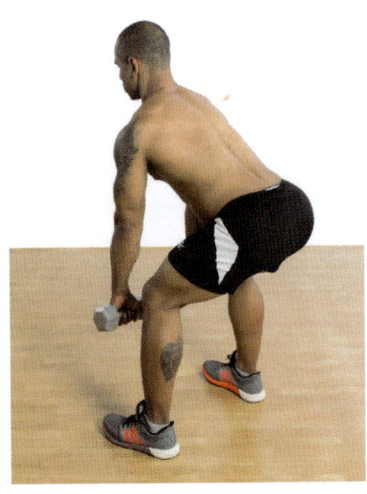

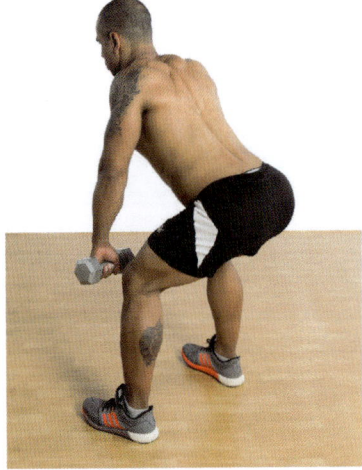

1. Stand in a bent-over position. Your arms should be fully extended with a dumbbell in each hand.

2. While maintaining straight arms, squeeze your shoulder blades together.

Release the shoulder blades back to the starting position.

UPPER BACK MUSCLES

Barbell Row

EQUIPMENT: Barbell

PRIME MOVERS: Rhomboids, middle trapezius, posterior deltoids

ASSISTANT MOVERS: Latissimus dorsi, biceps

STABILIZERS: Core muscles, quadriceps, hamstrings, forearm muscles

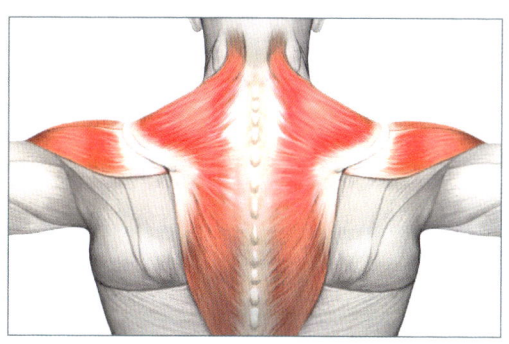

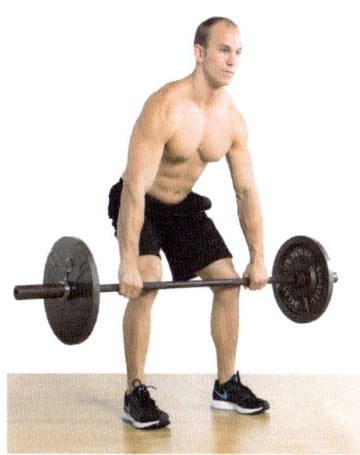

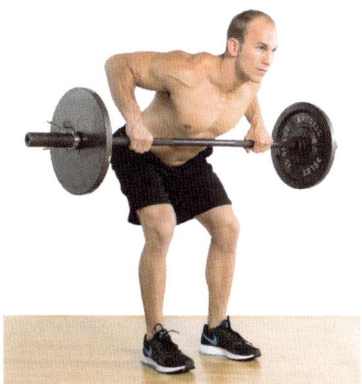

1. Stand in a bent over position. Your arms should be fully extended holding a barbell with your palms facing your body.

2. Squeeze your shoulder blades together and pull the bar up until it's close to touching the lower portion of your chest. Your elbows should be pointing out to the sides.

Lower the bar back to the starting position.

DELTOIDS (SHOULDERS)

The deltoid muscles act on the ball-and-socket shoulder joint in a variety of ways. The deltoids' three heads may act together, but they also have their own individual functions.

Muscles & Actions

The deltoid muscle is composed of three different heads, each performing different functions. When training the deltoids, it's important to be aware of which heads are working to produce a particular movement in order to get the desired training effect.

Anterior deltoid: Lateral adduction (specifically with external rotation) and forward extension of the humerus.

Lateral deltoid: Lateral abduction of the humerus.

Posterior deltoid: Lateral abduction of the humerus.

Training Tips

- When training the shoulders, it's important to utilize a diverse range of movements. Since the deltoids are responsible for so many movements, fully training them means choosing exercises that work the deltoids in every range of motion.

- When performing any deltoid exercise, try to maintain scapular retraction throughout the duration of the exercise.

- Avoid elevating your shoulders when performing deltoid exercises.

- Overhead movements may be dangerous if performed with improper form. Pay special attention to the instructions and terminate the exercise if you experience any problems.

- When possible, perform deltoid exercises with the palms in a neutral (parallel or facing each other) position to avoid shoulder impingement.

DELTOIDS (SHOULDERS) 33

Dumbbell Lateral Raise

EQUIPMENT: Dumbbells

PRIME MOVER: Deltoids (lateral)

ASSISTANT MOVER: Trapezius (upper portion)

STABILIZERS: Rotator cuff muscles, biceps, triceps, forearm muscles

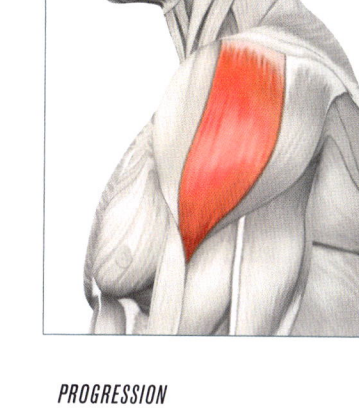

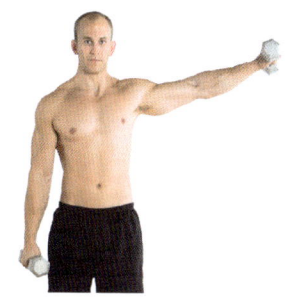

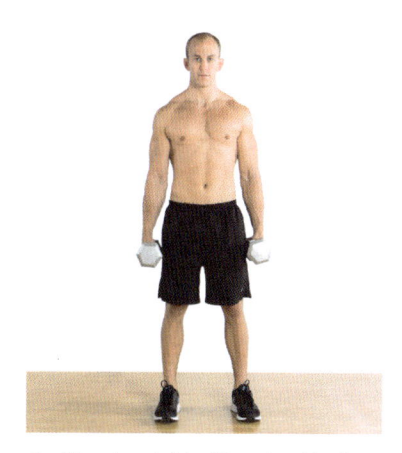

1. Stand upright with a dumbbell in each hand. Your palms should be in a neutral position and your elbows slightly bent.

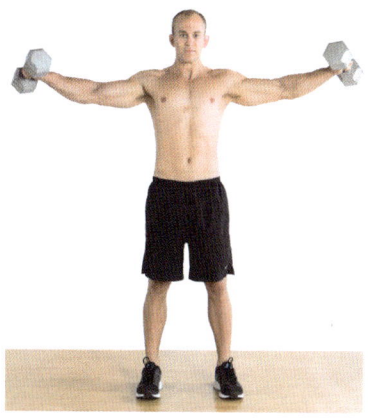

2. Maintaining the slight bend in your elbows, raise your arms until they're parallel to the floor.

Lower your arms back to the starting position.

PROGRESSION

- Begin with both arms extended out to the sides and perform all of the repetitions with one arm at a time.

REGRESSION

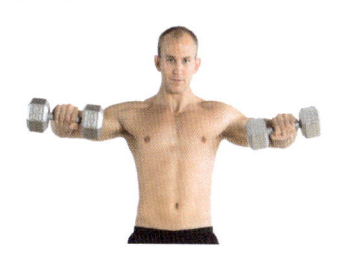

- Bending your elbows will decrease the difficulty of the exercise by shortening the lever. The more you bend your elbows, the easier this will be. Begin with your elbows bent at your sides and maintain the same angle throughout the movement.

NOTES

- Try not to raise your shoulders while you perform the movement.

Dumbbell Front Raise

EQUIPMENT: **Dumbbells**

PRIME MOVER: **Deltoids (anterior)**

ASSISTANT MOVER: **Trapezius**

STABILIZERS: **Rotator cuff muscles, biceps, triceps, forearm muscles**

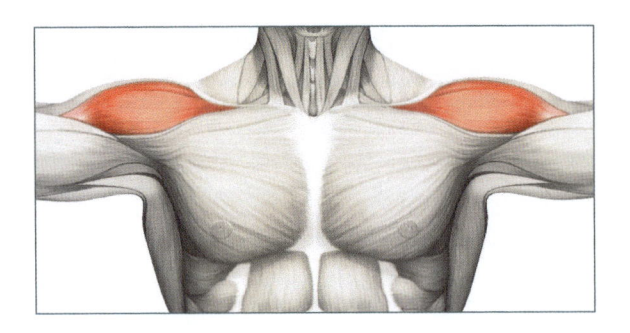

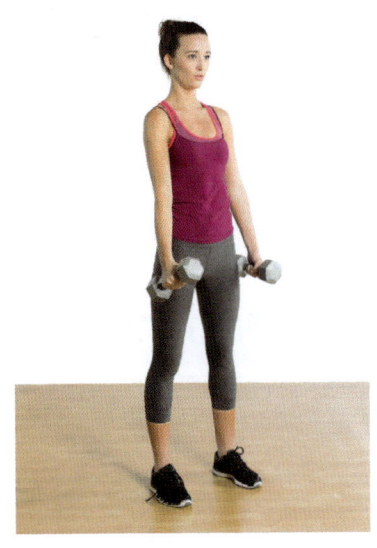

1. Stand upright with a dumbbell in each hand and your arms hanging in front of you. Your arms should be fully extended with your palms facing each other.

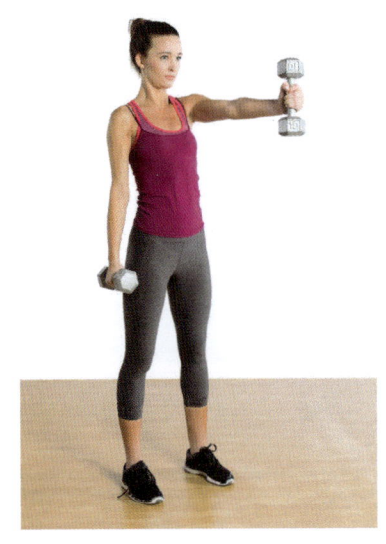

2. Using one arm at a time and maintaining the angle of your elbow, raise your arm up in front of you until your hand reaches eye level.

Lower back to the starting position.

NOTES

- When performing the exercise, bring your arm to a full stop before using the other arm.
- Performing this exercise with your palms down or facing your body can lead to shoulder impingement. It's recommended to perform this exercise with your palms in a neutral position.

DELTOIDS (SHOULDERS) 35

Shoulder Press

EQUIPMENT: Dumbbells

PRIME MOVERS: Deltoids (anterior, lateral)

ASSISTANT MOVERS: Triceps, trapezius

STABILIZERS: Core muscles, rotator cuff muscles

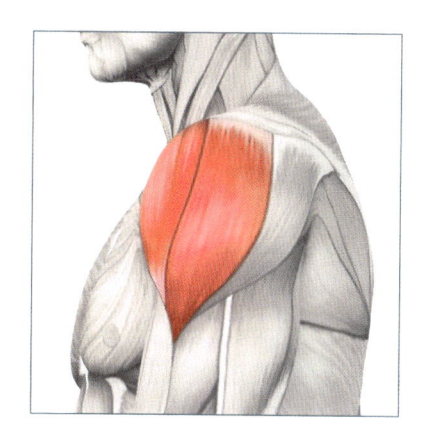

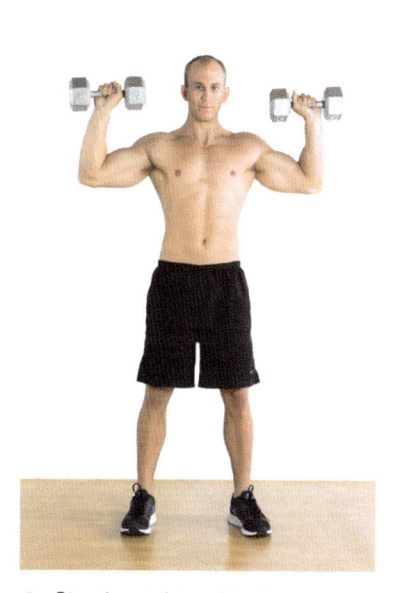

1. Stand upright and hold a dumbbell in each hand. Bend your elbows about 90 degrees and bring your upper arms (humerus) slightly below parallel to the floor (think cactus or goal posts).

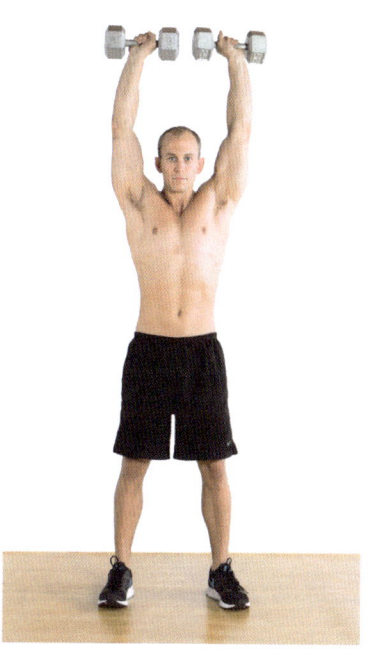

2. Press both arms up toward the ceiling until they're fully extended. The dumbbells should be 1 to 3 inches apart.

Trace the same arc back down to the starting position.

Upright Row

EQUIPMENT: **Barbell**

PRIME MOVERS: **Deltoids**

ASSISTANT MOVERS: Trapezius, biceps

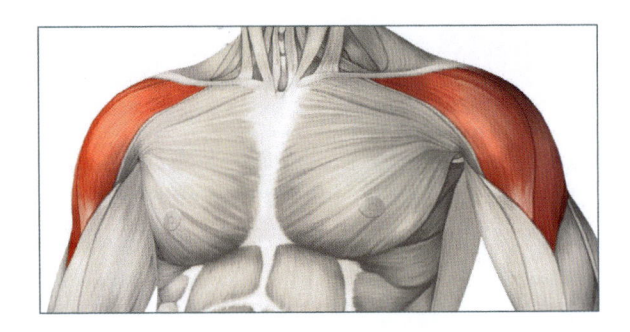

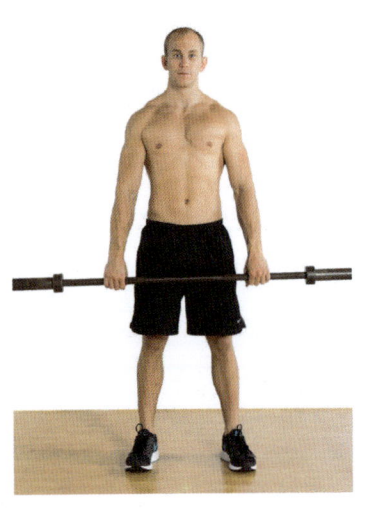

1. Stand upright holding a barbell in front of you with your hands shoulder-width apart and palms facing your thighs.

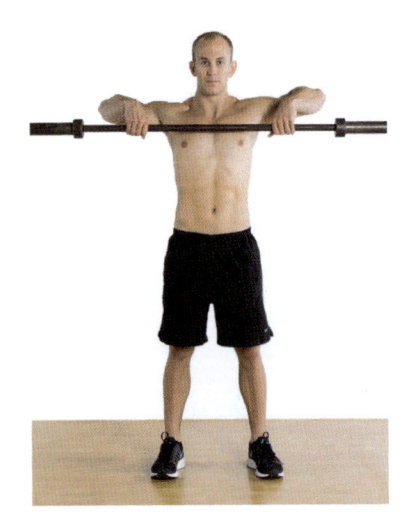

2. Moving your elbows out to the sides, pull the bar up until it's about chest level and your upper arm (humerus) is parallel to the floor.

Lower back to the starting position.

NOTES

- Don't raise your shoulders when performing this movement.
- Make sure that your elbows are always higher than the bar throughout the movement.

DELTOIDS (SHOULDERS) 37

Rear Deltoid Dumbbell Row

EQUIPMENT: Dumbbells

PRIME MOVER: Deltoids (posterior)

ASSISTANT MOVERS: Trapezius, rhomboids, forearm muscles

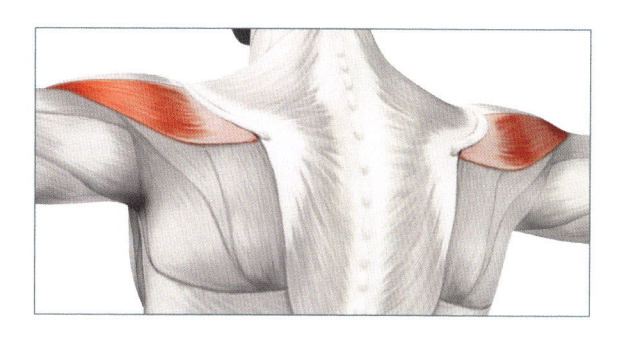

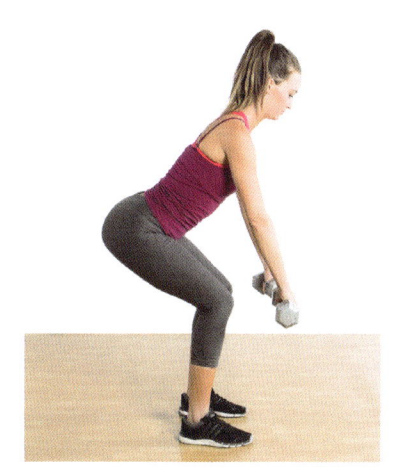

PROGRESSION

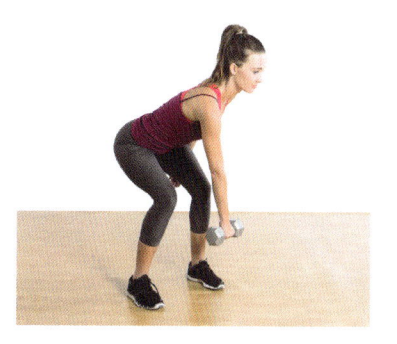

1. Stand in a bent-over position with a dumbbell in each hand and your palms facing your thighs. Your arms should be fully extended.

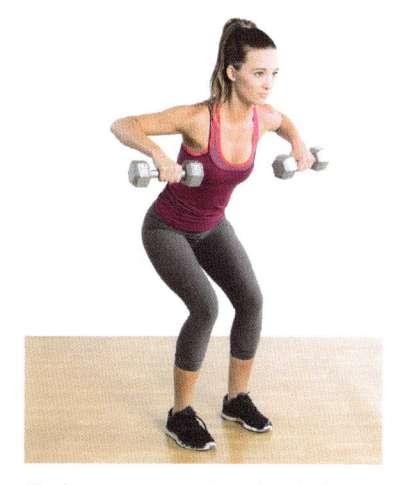

2. Squeeze your shoulder blades together and pull the dumbbells up until your upper arms are parallel to the floor and your elbows are out to the sides.

Lower back to the starting position.

- Using one dumbbell, begin with your arm across your chest past the middle of the body.

Dumbbell Reverse Fly

EQUIPMENT: **Dumbbells**

PRIME MOVER: **Deltoids (posterior)**

ASSISTANT MOVERS: **Trapezius, rhomboids**

STABILIZERS: **Core muscles, forearm muscles, biceps, triceps**

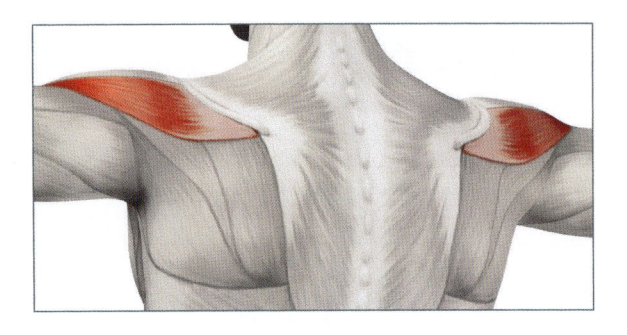

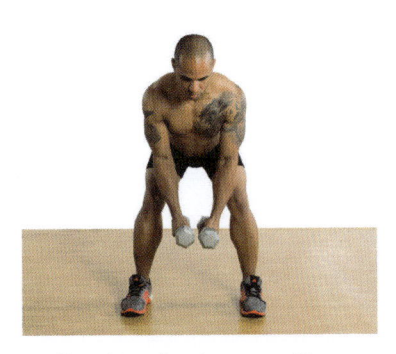

1. Stand in a bent-over position with a dumbbell in each hand and your palms facing each other. Your arms should be fully extended.

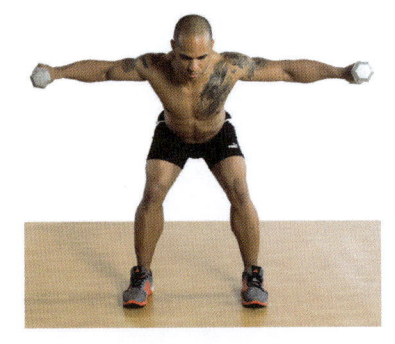

2. Maintaining straight arms, open your arms out to the sides until they're parallel to the floor.

Lower your arms back to the starting position.

PROGRESSION

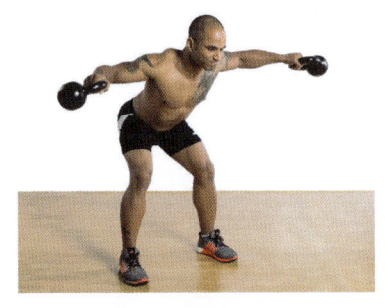

- Try this movement with kettlebells instead.

REGRESSION

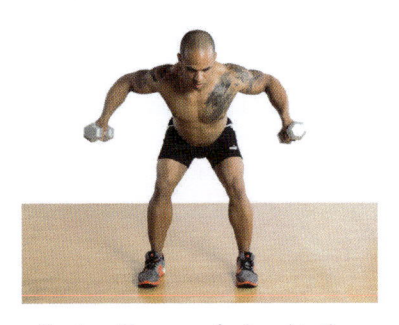

- Begin with more of a bend in the elbows and maintain the angle throughout the movement.

DELTOIDS (SHOULDERS) 39

Explosive Push Press

EQUIPMENT: Barbell
PRIME MOVERS: Deltoids
ASSISTANT MOVERS: Quadriceps, trapezius, triceps, calves
STABILIZERS: Core muscles, forearm muscles
PREREQUISITE EXERCISES: Shoulder press (page 35), barbell squat (page 70)

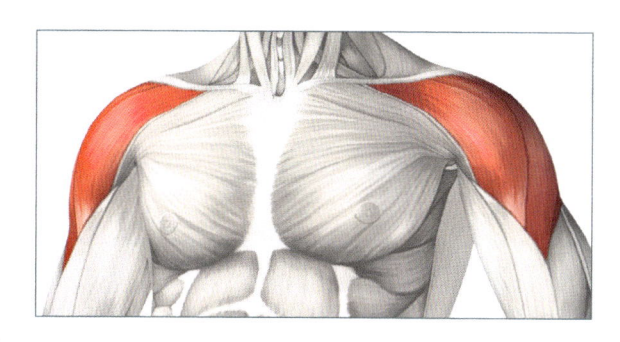

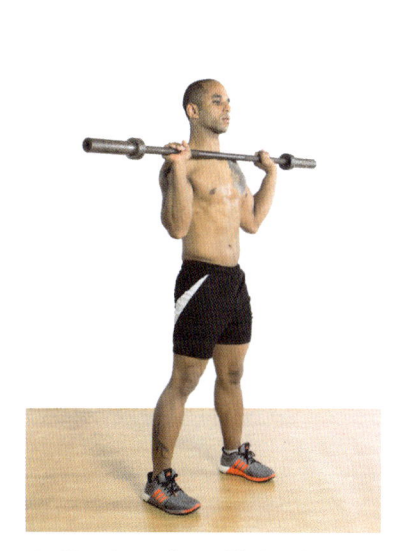

1. Stand upright and hold a barbell in both hands at your upper chest with your palms facing away from your body.

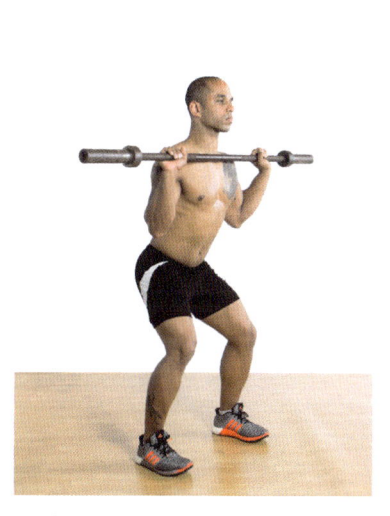

2. Sit back into a quarter squat.

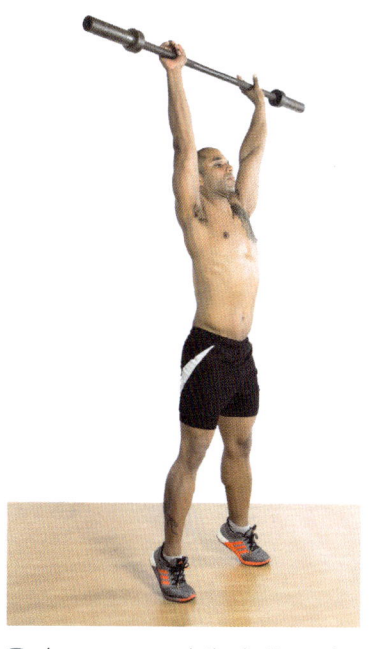

3. As you approach the bottom of the squat, immediately straighten your legs and use the momentum generated to assist you in pressing the bar overhead until your arms are fully extended. Your legs should be extended and, if necessary, your heels may come off the ground (calf plantarflexion).

As you lower the weight, bend your knees back into the quarter squat.

NOTES

- It's important to perform each repetition as quickly and powerfully as you can.

BICEPS

The biceps consist of muscles that connect the humerus (upper arm bone) to the shoulder as well as to the lower part of the arm (radius and ulna). They work primarily to flex the elbow but assist in a variety of other movements.

Muscles & Actions

Biceps brachii: Composed of a long and a short head, the biceps brachii flex the elbow as well as supinate the forearm. They also assist in forward shoulder extension.

Brachialis: The brachialis is actually the strongest flexor of the elbow.

Brachioradialis: This muscle assists in flexing the elbow.

Training Tips

- The biceps brachii act on three joints (the shoulder, the elbow, the radioulnar), so any exercise program should include a variety of movements that use the biceps to act on the different joints.

- The brachialis, which is the strongest elbow flexor, should not be overlooked when training. Elbow flexion with your palms in a neutral position is great for working the brachialis.

- Injuries to the biceps tendon are common, so avoid full extension, especially with heavier weights.

BICEPS 41

Dumbbell Biceps Curl

EQUIPMENT: Dumbbells

PRIME MOVERS: Brachialis, biceps brachii

ASSISTANT MOVERS: Brachioradialis, supinator

STABILIZERS: Rotator cuff muscles, rhomboids, forearm muscles

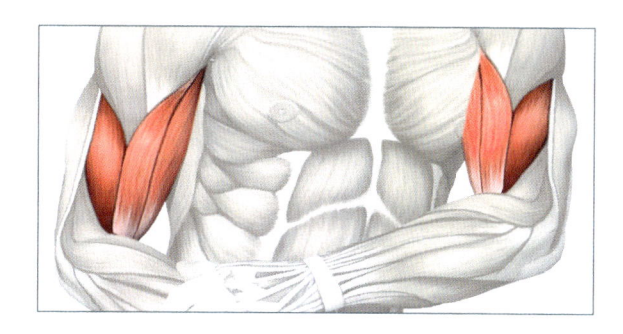

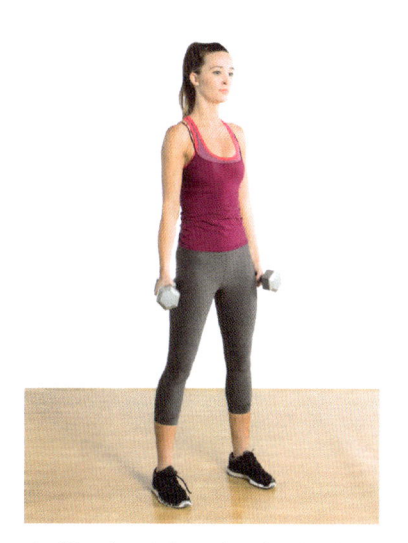

PROGRESSION

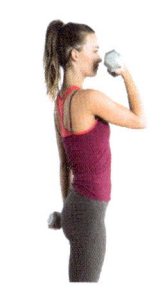

1. Stand upright with a dumbbell in each hand and your arms hanging by your sides. Your palms should be in a neutral position, facing each other.

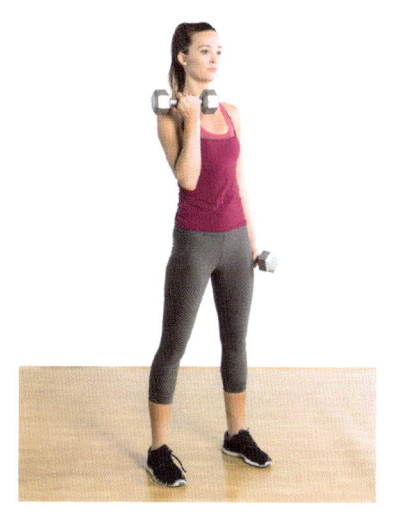

2. Alternating arms, in one motion, turn your palm up while simultaneously bringing the dumbbell in line with your shoulder.

Lower back to the starting position.

- Add slight flexion at your shoulder by lifting your arm as you perform the curl.

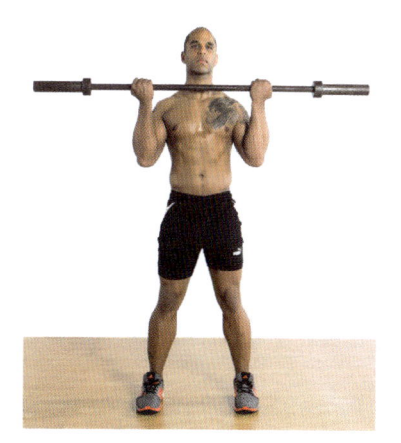

- This can also be done with a barbell. Be careful not to overextend your lower back.

Dumbbell Hammer Curl

EQUIPMENT: **Dumbbells**

PRIME MOVER: **Brachialis**

ASSISTANT MOVERS: **Biceps brachii, brachioradialis**

STABILIZERS: **Rotator cuff muscles, rhomboids, forearm muscles**

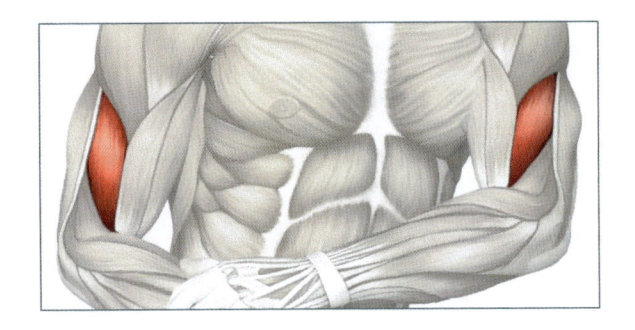

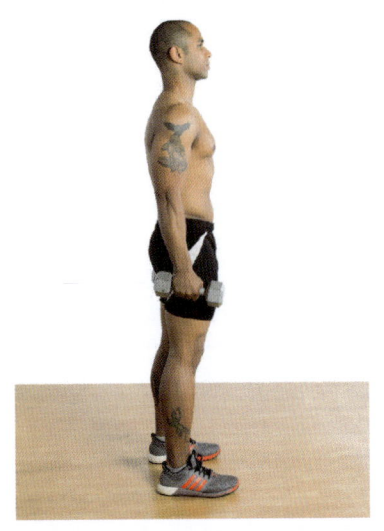

1. Stand upright with a dumbbell in each hand and your palms facing each other.

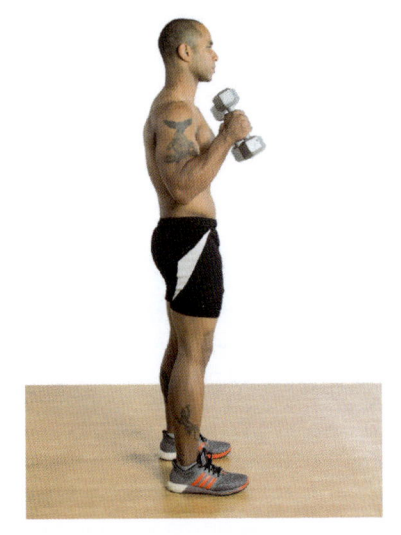

2. Bend your elbows until the dumbbells are in line with your shoulders.

Lower back to the starting position.

Kettlebell Kneeling Concentration Curl

EQUIPMENT: Kettlebell

PRIME MOVERS: Brachialis, biceps brachii

ASSISTANT MOVERS: Brachioradialis, supinator

STABILIZERS: Rotator cuff muscles, rhomboids, forearm muscles

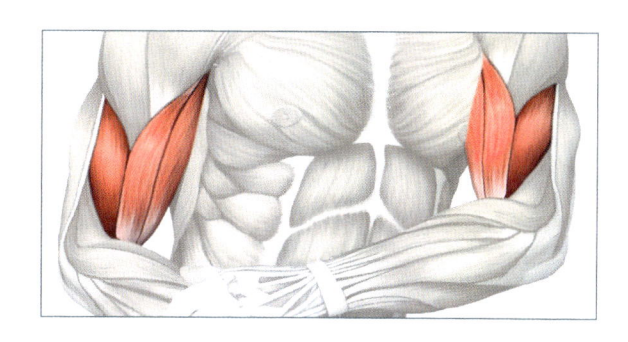

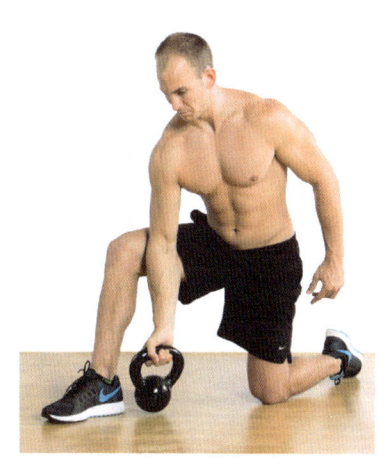

PROGRESSION

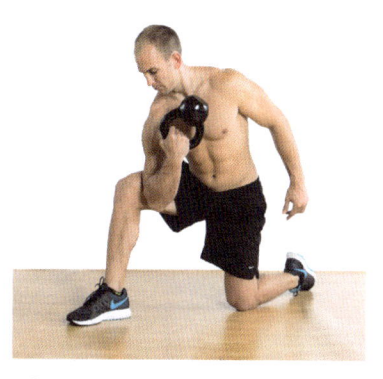

1. Kneel with your left knee and right foot on the floor. Your right upper arm should be placed on your inner thigh with a kettlebell in your hand.

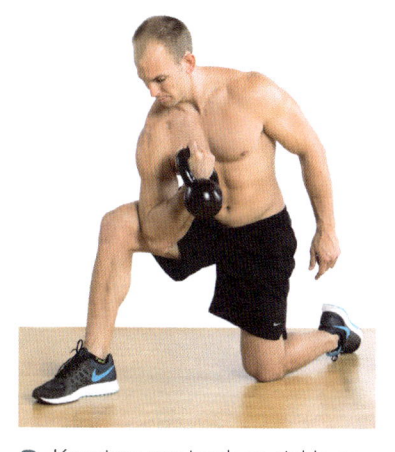

2. Keeping your trunk as stable as possible throughout the movement, flex your elbow to bring the kettlebell up.

Control back down to the starting position.

- Stabilize the kettlebell so that the bottom is pointing up toward the ceiling at the top of the movement.

TRICEPS

The large muscle on the back of the upper arm, the triceps are a three-headed muscle that acts on the elbow and the shoulder.

Muscles & Actions

Triceps: Composed of three heads (long, medial, lateral), the triceps extend the elbow and also assist in the adduction of the humerus (upper arm bone). All three heads perform the same function, with slight differences in which head is emphasized during exercise. Arms down to the side and palms down will place slightly more emphasis on the medial head. Arms down to the side and palms up will place slightly more emphasis on the lateral head. Arms extended forward or overhead will place slightly more emphasis on the long head.

Training Tips

- In order to properly train the triceps, it's important to maintain stability in the shoulders and only move at the elbow joint.

- When performing exercises that do involve movement at the shoulders, keep your arms close to your torso.

TRICEPS 45

Bench Dip

EQUIPMENT: None
PRIME MOVERS: Triceps
ASSISTANT MOVERS: Deltoids
STABILIZERS: Core muscles, quadriceps

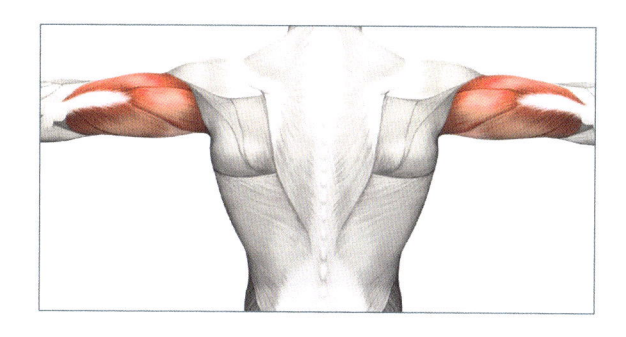

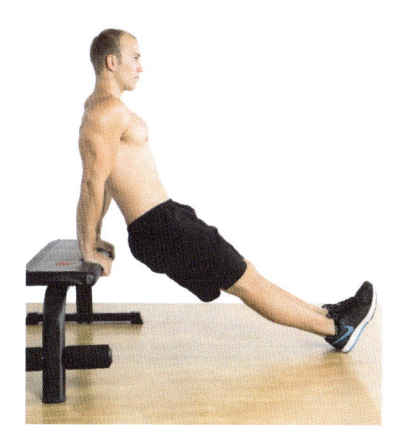

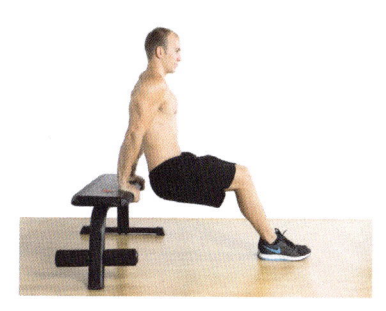

REGRESSION

- Bend your knees.

1. Sit on the edge of a bench with your arms directly by your sides and your hands on either side of you on the bench, fingers facing forward. Your legs should be fully extended with your heels touching the floor. Lift yourself off of the bench.

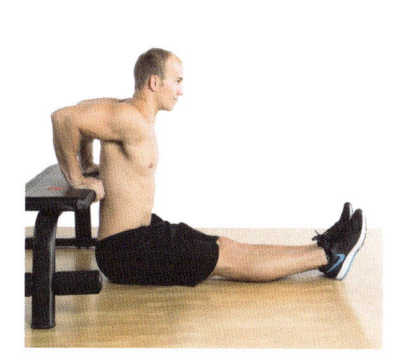

2. Keeping your back straight and torso perpendicular to the floor, bend your elbows straight back and lower yourself toward the floor as low as you can comfortably get.

Straighten your elbows back to the starting position.

NOTES
- This can be a difficult exercise if you have any deltoid or rotator cuff injuries.

Dumbbell Kickback

EQUIPMENT: **Dumbbells**

PRIME MOVERS: **Triceps**

STABILIZERS: **Rotator cuff muscles, rhomboids, trapezius, forearm muscles**

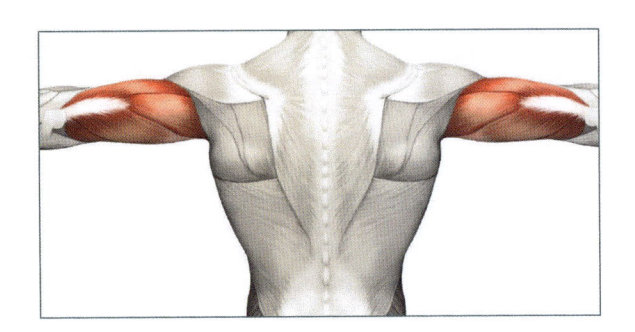

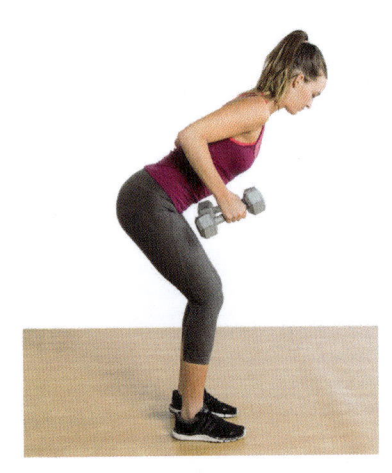

1. Stand in a bent-over position with a dumbbell in each hand. Your upper arms should be next to and in line with your torso and your elbows bent.

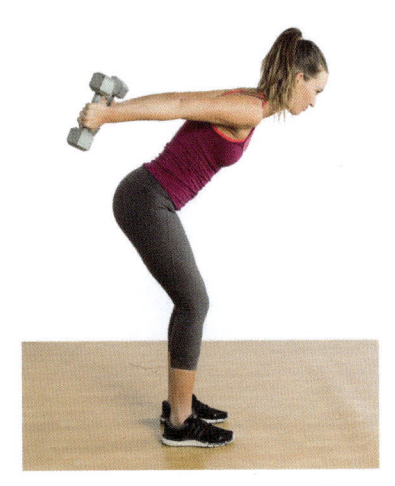

2. Straighten both elbows until your arms are fully extended.

Return to the starting position.

TRICEPS 47

Bent-Over T Extension

EQUIPMENT: Dumbbells

PRIME MOVERS: Triceps

STABILIZERS: Deltoids, trapezius, rhomboids, forearm muscles

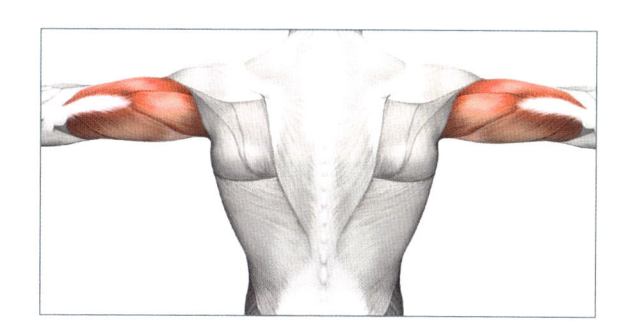

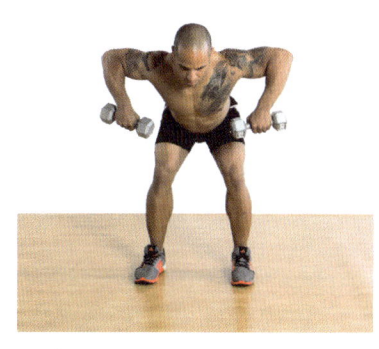

1. Stand in a bent-over position with a dumbbell in each hand. Bend your elbows and bring them out to the sides and in line with your shoulders.

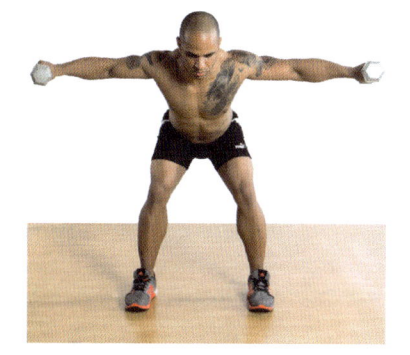

2. Maintaining a stable shoulder position throughout the movement, extend your elbows until your arms are fully extended and form a "T" with your torso.

Bend your elbows back to the starting position.

Close-Grip Bench Press

EQUIPMENT: Barbell

PRIME MOVERS: Triceps

ASSISTANT MOVERS: Deltoids, pectoralis major

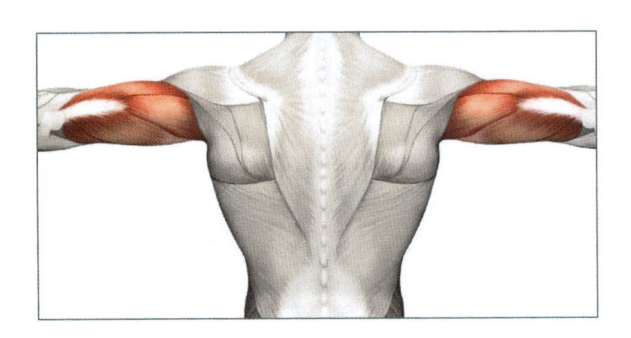

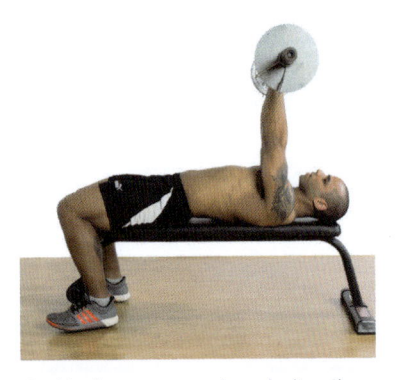

1. Lie face-up on a bench directly under a barbell. Grip the bar with your hands slightly narrower than shoulder-width apart.

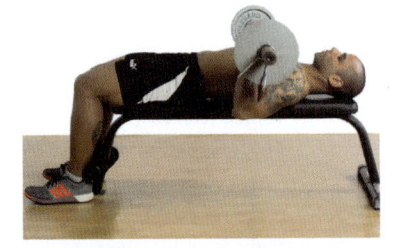

2. Keeping your upper arms close to your body instead of letting your elbows flare out to the sides, lower the bar toward your chest until it's 2 to 6 inches above the lower portion of your chest.

Press the weight back up to the starting position.

Kettlebell Triceps Extension

EQUIPMENT: Kettlebell

PRIME MOVERS: Triceps

STABILIZERS: Deltoids, rotator cuff muscles, forearm muscles

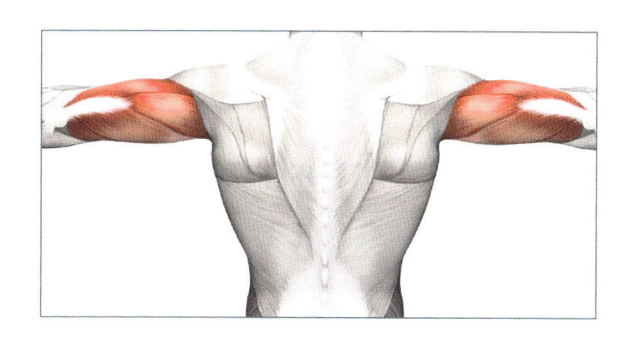

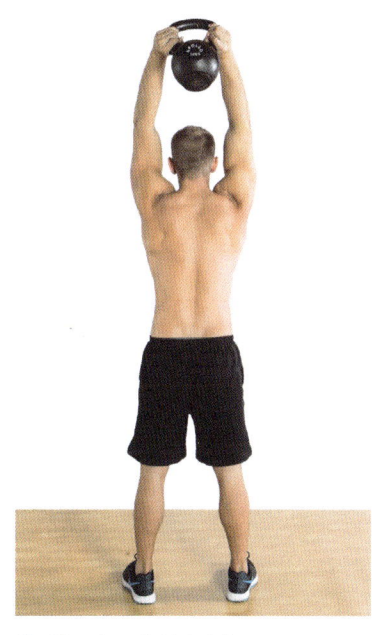

1. Stand upright holding one kettlebell in both hands. Grip the outside of the handle with your palms facing each other and extend both arms toward the ceiling.

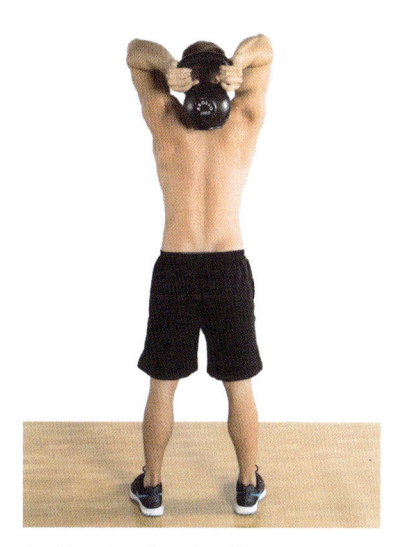

2. Keeping the shoulder position and maintaining stable shoulders throughout the movement, bend both elbows and lower the kettlebell behind you as far back as you comfortably can.

Extend both arms back to the starting position.

NOTES

- This can be a difficult exercise if you have and deltoid or rotator cuff injuries.

TRUNK MUSCLES

The trunk muscles consist of the core, abdominals, lower back, and hip flexors. While these muscles are grouped together, it's important to understand the difference between them in order to properly train the trunk. When training the abdominals and lower back, the focus is on muscles that flex, laterally flex, and extend the trunk. When training the hip flexors, the focus is on the muscles that flex the femur (upper leg bone). When training the core, the focus is on engaging the muscles that stabilize the spine and pelvis.

Muscles & Actions

ABDOMINALS

Rectus abdominis: The long muscle on the front of the trunk (often identified as the six-pack muscle), this flexes the lumbar spine and helps to develop intra-abdominal pressure.

External oblique: The long muscle found on either side of the trunk, this assists in flexion and rotation of the spine; one side can work to produce lateral flexion. It also works to produce intra-abdominal pressure.

Internal oblique: A deeper muscle than the external oblique and found on either side of the trunk, this assists in flexion, lateral flexion, and rotation of the spine. It works together with the external oblique to produce lateral flexion and rotation. All three muscles work together to produce trunk flexion.

LOWER BACK

Erector spinae: Muscles along the back of the trunk on either side of the spine.

Iliocostalis: Assists in spinal extension and lateral flexion.

Longissimus: Assists in spinal extension and lateral flexion.

Spinalis: Assists in extension of the thoracic spine.

Multifidus: Assists in rotation, lateral flexion, and extension of the spine.

HIP FLEXORS

Psoas major: Attaching at the femur and the lumbar spine, this assists in hip flexion, lateral flexion, and extension of the lumbar spine.

Psoas minor: Attaching at the pelvic bone and the lumbar spine, this assists in flexion of the spine.

Iliacus: Attaching at the pelvic bone and the femur, this assists in flexion and external rotation of the thigh.

Pectineus: Attaching at the pelvic bone and the femur, this assists in flexion, adduction, and internal rotation of the thigh.

CORE MUSCLES

Transverse abdominis (TVA): A belt-like muscle on the lower half of the trunk, this compresses the ribs to assist with trunk stabilization.

Quadratus lumborum (QL): Connecting at the pelvic bone as well as the lower rib, this assists in lateral flexion, lumbar stabilization, and extension of the lumbar spine.

Rectus abdominis: The long muscle on the front of the trunk (often identified as the six-pack muscle), this flexes the lumbar spine and helps to develop intra-abdominal pressure.

External oblique: The long muscle found on either side of the trunk, this assists in flexion and rotation of the spine; one side can work to produce lateral flexion. It also works to produce intra-abdominal pressure.

Internal oblique: A deeper muscle than the external oblique and found on either side of the trunk, this assists in flexion, lateral flexion, and rotation of the spine. It works together with the external oblique to produce lateral flexion and rotation. All three muscles work together to produce trunk flexion.

Erector spinae: Muscles along the back of the trunk on either side of the spine.

Training Tips

- When performing exercises that require a stable spine, engage your abdominals as if bracing for a punch.
- Contrary to what many magazines and trainers may say, there's no significant difference between the upper and lower abs. Further, leg raises, which are often stressed as a "lower abdominal exercise," are actually a hip flexor exercise.
- When performing leg raises and similar exercises, maintain a stable trunk and avoid overarching the lower back in order to develop the core and avoid injury.

Sit-Up

EQUIPMENT: None

PRIME MOVER: Rectus abdominis

ASSISTANT MOVERS: Internal and external obliques, psoas major

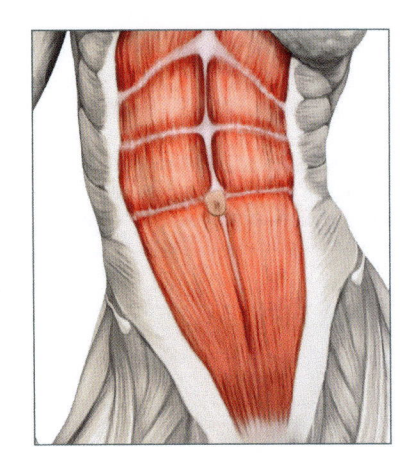

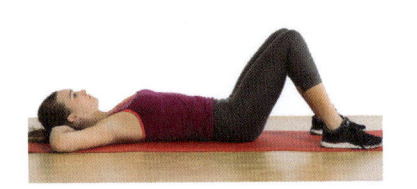

1. Lie face-up with your knees bent and feet on the floor. Your hands can be interlocked behind your head.

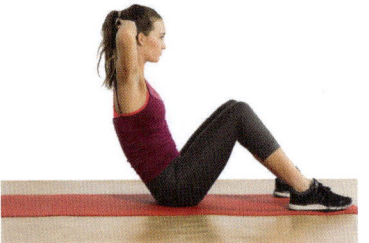

2. Squeeze your abdominals and curl your trunk upward until you're sitting up as high as you can.

Slowly lower back to the starting position.

PROGRESSION

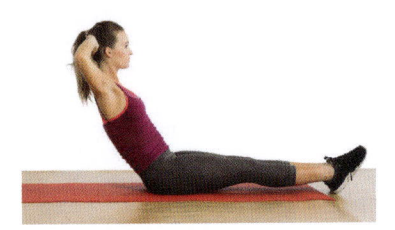

- Start with your legs completely straight.

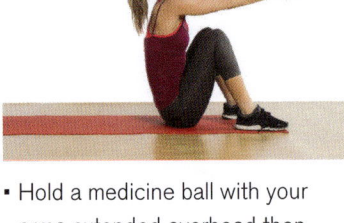

- Hold a medicine ball with your arms extended overhead then explosively swing your arms forward and sit up using the momentum from the swing to assist you.

REGRESSION

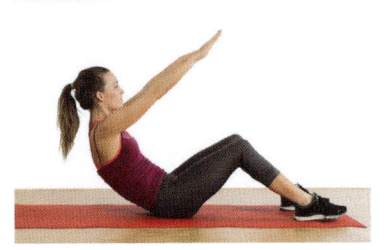

- Use your arms by swinging them up as you begin the movement.

NOTES

- On the way back to the starting position, make sure to engage your core and control yourself back down.

Crossover Crunch

EQUIPMENT: None

PRIME MOVERS: Internal and external obliques, rectus abdominis

ASSISTANT MOVER: Multifidus

STABILIZER: Hip flexor muscles

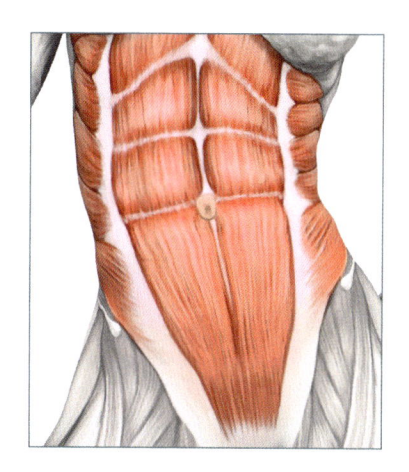

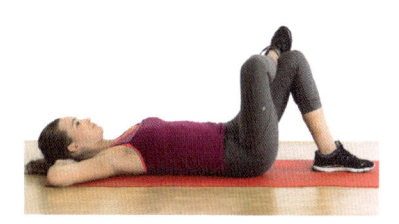

1. Lie face-up with your knees bent and feet on the floor. Place your right ankle across your left knee with your right knee extended out to the side. Place both hands behind your neck with your elbows out to the sides.

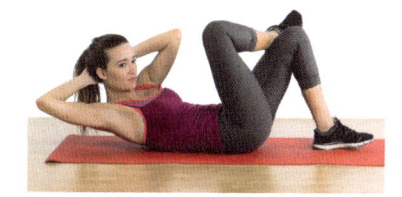

2. Keeping your elbows extended to the sides the entire time, curl your torso while simultaneously rotating to your right, moving your left elbow toward your right knee.

Lower back to the starting position.

Total-Body Crunch

EQUIPMENT: None

PRIME MOVER: Rectus abdominis

ASSISTANT MOVERS: Internal and external obliques, psoas major

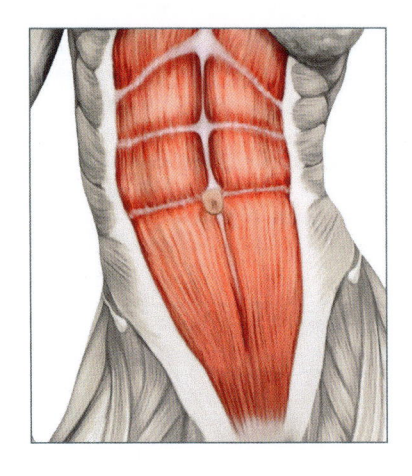

PROGRESSION

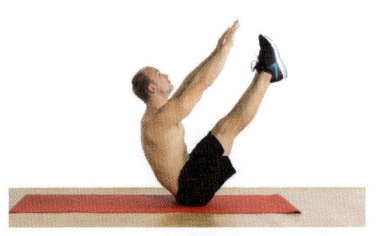

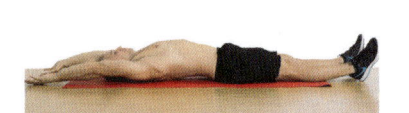

1. Lie face-up with your legs extended and your arms fully extended behind you.

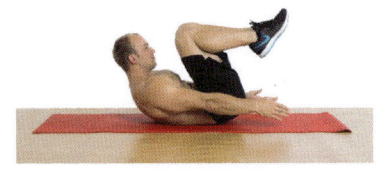

2. Swing your arms forward and curl up while simultaneously curling your knees into your chest. At the top of the movement, your arms should be at your sides with your shoulders 3 to 6 inches off of the floor. Your knees should be touching your chest.

Extend back to the starting position.

- Maintain straight legs throughout the movement and sit up fully until your body forms a "V."

Medicine Ball Seated Rotation

EQUIPMENT: Medicine ball

PRIME MOVERS: Internal and external obliques

ASSISTANT MOVERS: Rectus abdominis, multifidus

STABILIZERS: Transverse abdominis, rectus abdominis, hip flexor muscles, quadriceps

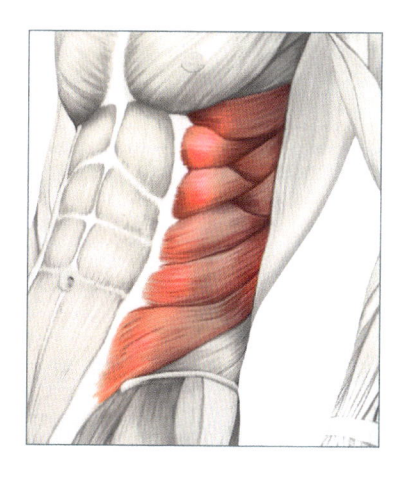

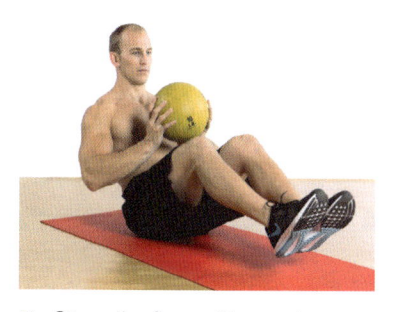

1. Sit on the floor with your torso leaning back up to 45 degrees, your legs slightly flexed, and your heels 6 inches off of the floor. Hold a medicine ball in front of you.

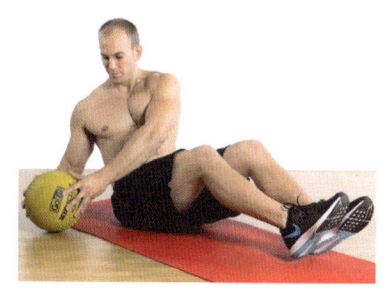

2. Rotate to one side and lower the medicine ball until you lightly touch the floor.

Quickly rotate in the opposite direction and repeat.

PROGRESSION

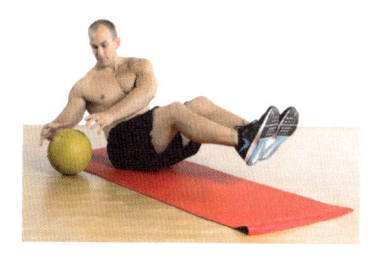

- Drop and catch the medicine ball on each side.

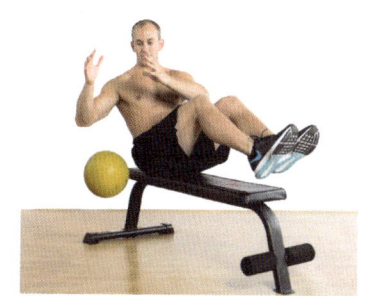

- Perform the exercise seated on an elevated surface like a step or a bench. Throw and catch the medicine ball.

Medicine Ball Wraparound

EQUIPMENT: Medicine ball
PRIME MOVERS: Quadriceps, internal and external obliques
ASSISTANT MOVERS: Calves, gluteal muscles, deltoids
STABILIZERS: Biceps, triceps

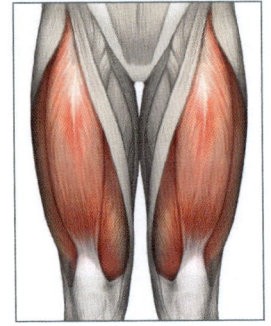

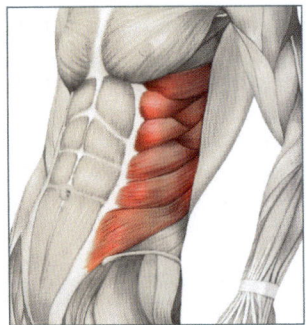

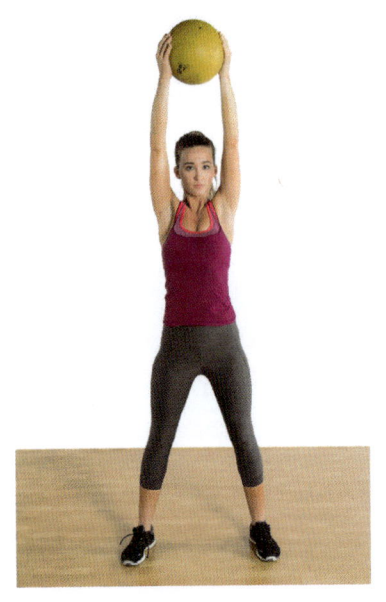

1. Stand upright and hold a medicine ball overhead with your arms fully extended.

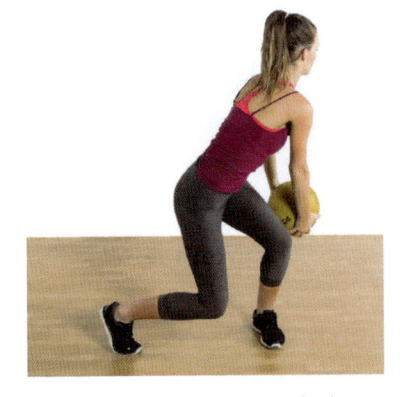

2. Keeping your torso upright, lower the medicine ball to your left and simultaneously bend your knees and pivot on your toes (especially your left). At the bottom of the movement, both knees should be flexed with your left leg rotated, pivoting on your toes. Your arms should be straight, holding the medicine ball outside of your left leg.

Maintaining straight arms, straighten both legs and wrap the medicine ball around back to the starting position. Repeat on the other side.

NOTES
- Once you're comfortable with the movement, move from side to side without pausing at the top of the movement.

Physioball Crunch

EQUIPMENT: Physioball

PRIME MOVER: Rectus abdominis

ASSISTANT MOVERS: Internal and external obliques

STABILIZERS: Hip flexor muscles, quadriceps

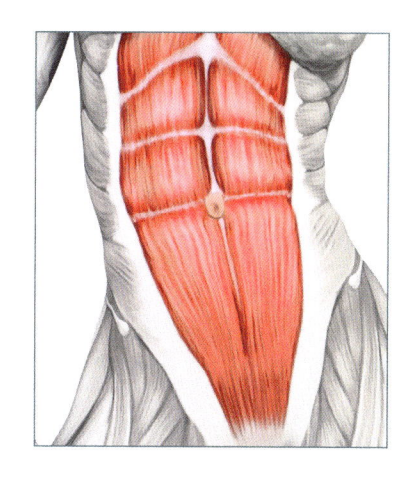

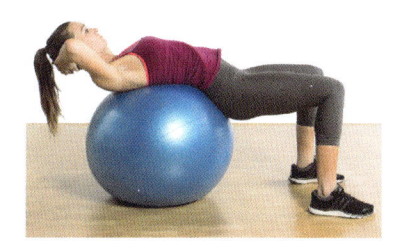

PROGRESSION
- Sit higher on the ball before performing the crunch.

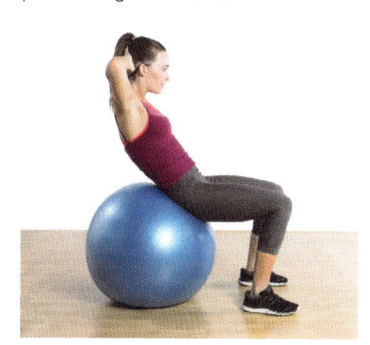

1. Lie with the middle of your lower back on a physioball. Your feet should be flat on the floor and hip-width apart. Interlock your hands behind your neck.

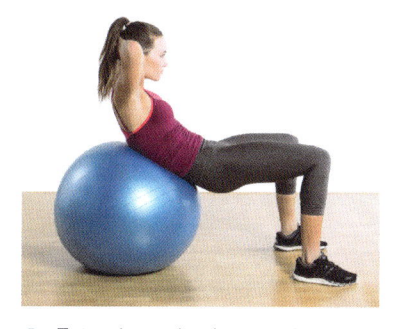

2. Extend your back around the ball as far as you comfortably can.

Curl back up, bringing your sternum to your pelvis.

Kettlebell Sit-Up

EQUIPMENT: Kettlebell

PRIME MOVERS: Rectus abdominis, psoas major

ASSISTANT MOVERS: Internal and external obliques

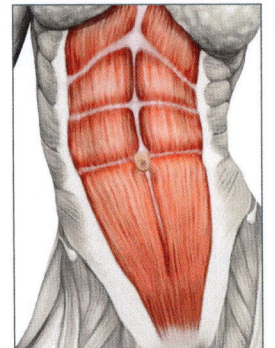

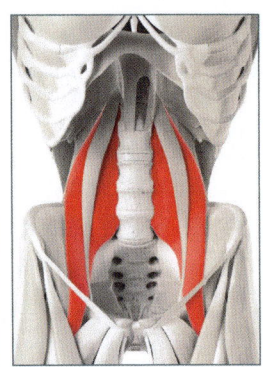

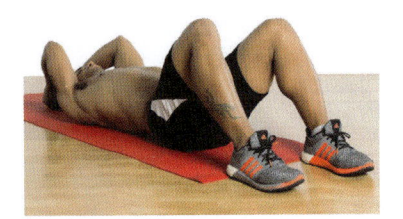

1. Lie face-up with your knees bent and feet on the floor. Hold a kettlebell in both hands and extend your arms overhead.

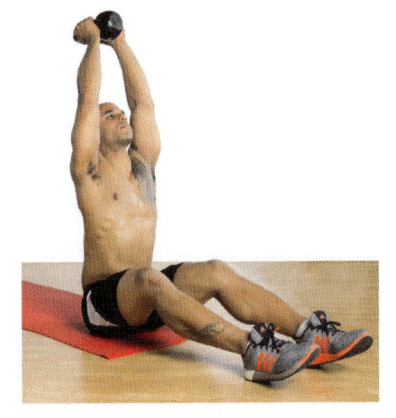

2. Explosively swing your arms forward and use the momentum of the arm swing to lift your torso off of the ground. As you approach the top, straighten out your torso and extend your arms toward the ceiling.

Slowly lower back to the starting position.

TRUNK MUSCLES

Superman

EQUIPMENT: None

PRIME MOVER: Erector spinae

ASSISTANT MOVERS: Multifidus, quadratus lumborum

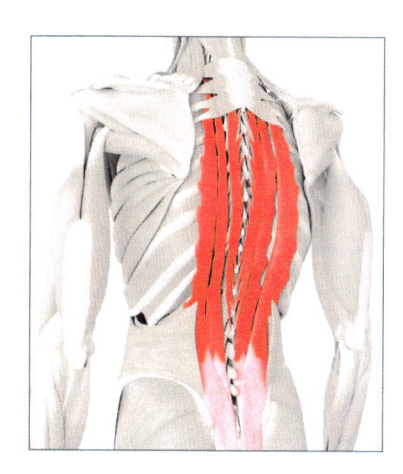

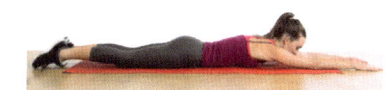

1. Lie facedown on the floor with your arms forward and your legs extended.

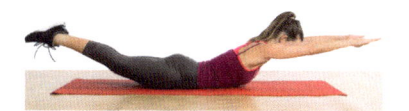

2. Extend your lumbar spine, lifting your legs and hips off of the floor. At the same time, lift your chest and arms off of the floor.

Lower back to the starting position.

Plank

EQUIPMENT: None

PRIME MOVERS: Core muscles

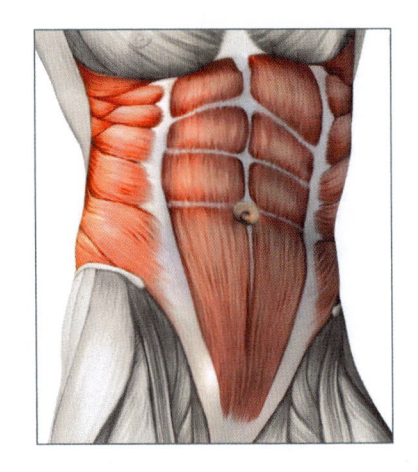

PROGRESSION

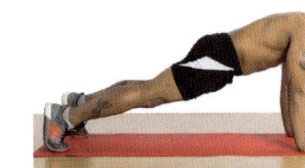

REGRESSION

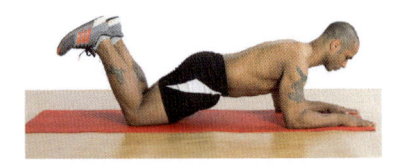

1. Lie facedown with your forearms flat on the floor, elbows bent 90 degrees, and your upper arms perpendicular to the floor. The points of contact should be your forearms and toes. Your trunk should be in a neutral position and your legs straight. This position should be maintained for a predetermined amount of time.

- Hold the position with straight arms.

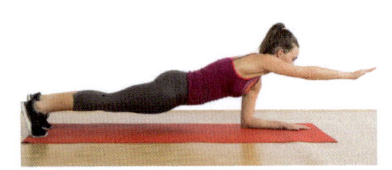

- Maintaining stability throughout your body, extend one arm and touch the floor in front of you. Pull your arm back and extend the opposite arm.

- Hold the position with your knees on the floor.

NOTES

- Maintain a stable trunk and try not to overarch.

TRUNK MUSCLES

Side Plank

EQUIPMENT: None

PRIME MOVERS: Internal and external obliques

ASSISTANT MOVERS: Core muscles

STABILIZERS: Gluteal muscles, quadriceps, hamstrings

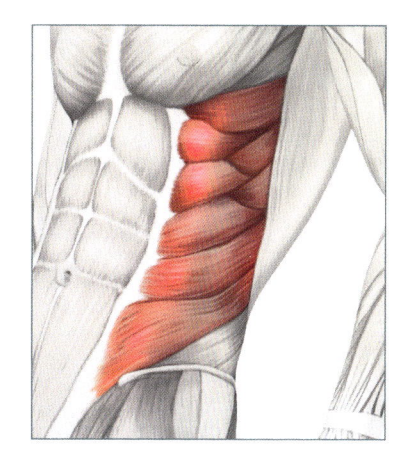

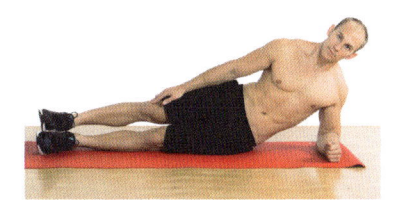

1. Lie on your side with your forearm, hip, and foot on the floor and in line with each other. Stack your hips, shoulders, and feet.

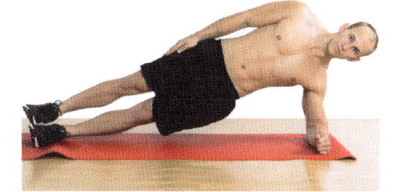

2. Maintaining a straight and stable torso, lift your hips off of the floor as high as you comfortably can. Make sure that your torso and trunk are in line.

Lower back to the starting position.

PROGRESSION

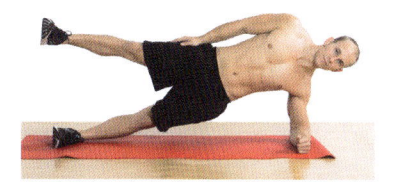

- Lift the top leg off of the bottom leg.

REGRESSION

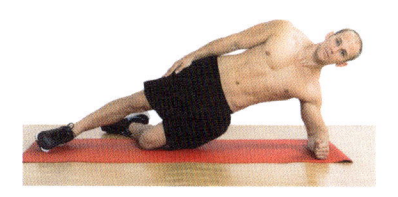

- If balance is an issue, bend your bottom knee and touch it to the floor.

Physioball Plank with Arm Extension

EQUIPMENT: **Physioball**

PRIME MOVERS: **Anterior deltoids, latissimus dorsi**

STABILIZERS: **Core muscles, quadriceps, upper back muscles**

PREREQUISITE EXERCISE: **Plank (page 60)**

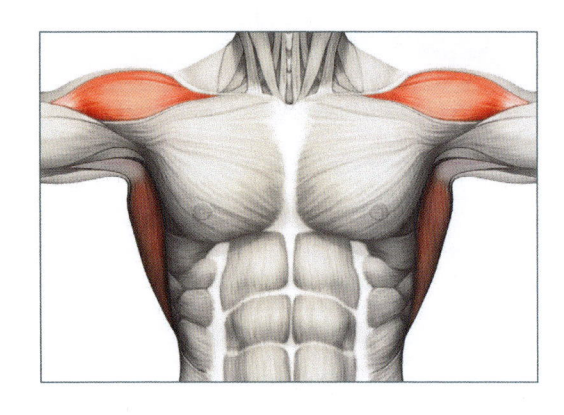

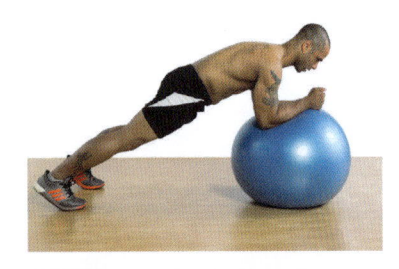

1. Place your forearms on the physioball and assume a plank position.

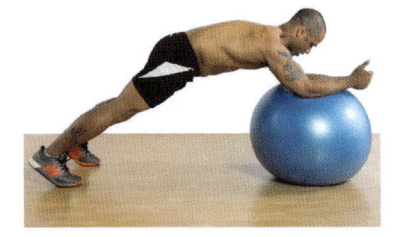

2. Extend your arms from the shoulders as far as you comfortably can.

At the middle of the movement, your trunk should remain parallel to the floor and in a neutral position. Your arms should be extended at the shoulders with your forearms on the ball. The ball should roll underneath your forearms.

Kneeling Rollout

EQUIPMENT: Physioball

PRIME MOVER: Latissimus dorsi

ASSISTANT MOVERS: Pectoralis minor, serratus anterior

STABILIZERS: Core muscles, biceps, triceps

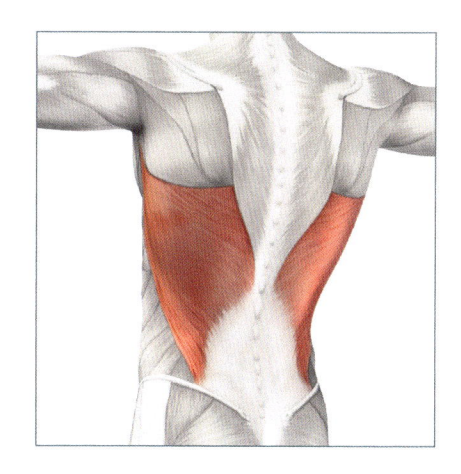

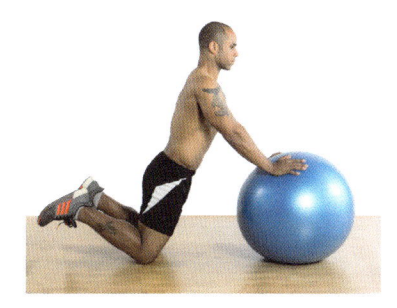

1. Kneel on the floor with your hands on a physioball and arms fully extended. Your feet should be off of the floor behind you. There should be a straight line between your knees and shoulders as well as your shoulders and hands. Pivoting on your knees, shift your weight forward so that your weight is on the ball.

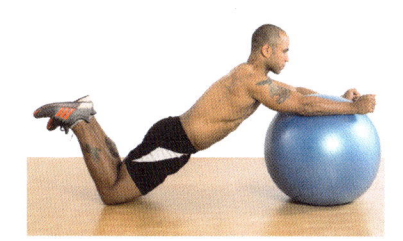

2. Roll forward so that the ball moves onto your forearms. Maintain a stable core as well as the extension in your arms and at your waist. Remember to pivot on your knees. Pause at the end of the movement.

Roll back to the starting position.

NOTES
- The movement should occur only at your shoulders. Maintain a straight back and arms throughout the movement.

Seated Kettlebell Toss

EQUIPMENT: **Kettlebell**

PRIME MOVERS: **Core muscles**

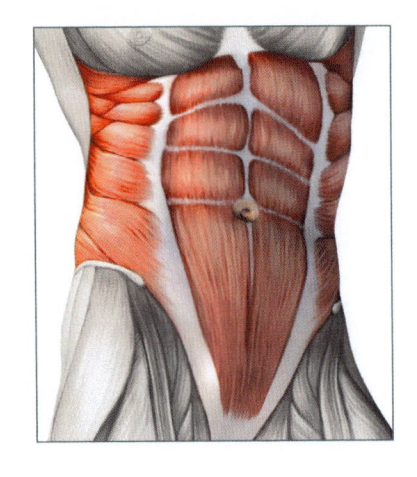

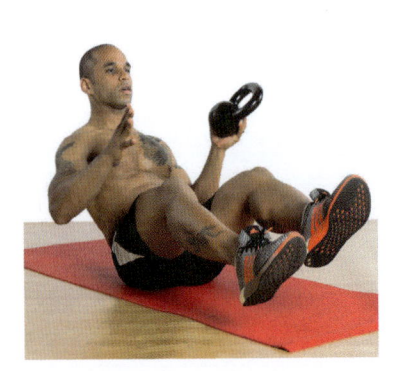

1. Sit on the floor with your legs extended. Lift your heels off of the floor and lean your torso back slightly, maintaining a straight and stable spine. Keeping your arms bent and 8 to 16 inches apart, in one hand hold a kettlebell from the bottom.

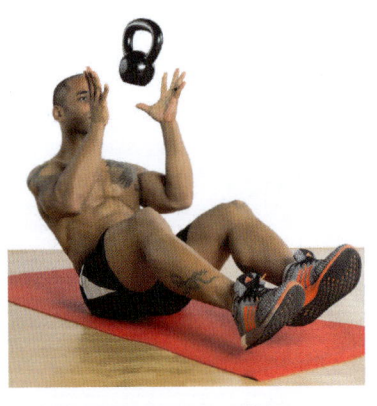

2. Maintaining your position throughout the exercise, toss the kettlebell side to side.

PROGRESSION

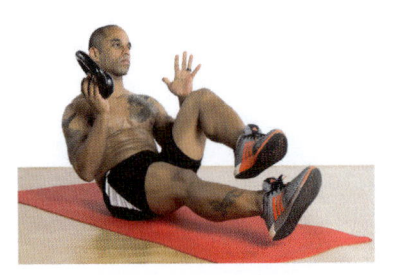

- Add bicycle kicks to the toss by alternatively pulling one knee in and fully extending the other one with each toss.

Leg Lowering

EQUIPMENT: None

PRIME MOVERS: Hip flexor muscles

ASSISTANT MOVERS: Quadriceps, psoas major

STABILIZERS: Core muscles

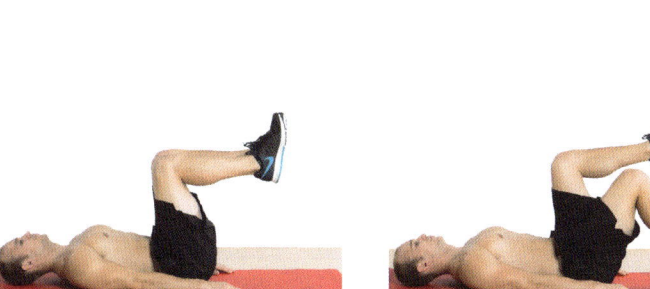

1. Lie face-up and lift both legs so that your hips and knees are bent 90 degrees.

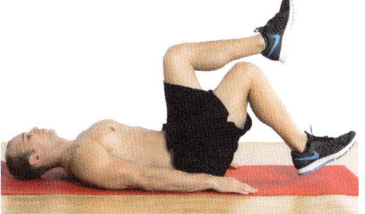

2. Maintaining the angle at the knee throughout the movement and bracing your abdominals, lower one leg from the hips until your heel lightly touches the floor.

Raise your leg back to the starting position.

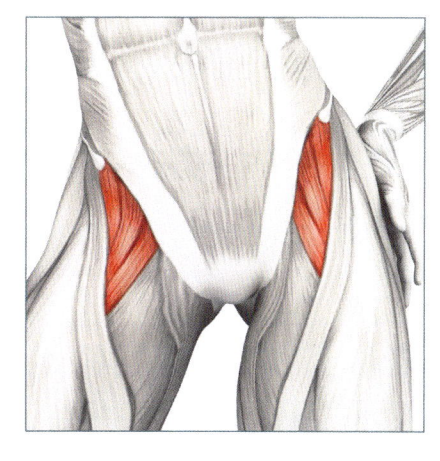

PROGRESSION

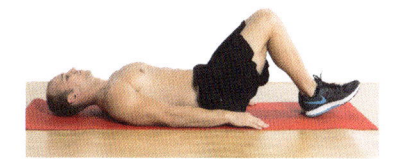

- Lower both legs at the same time.

REGRESSION

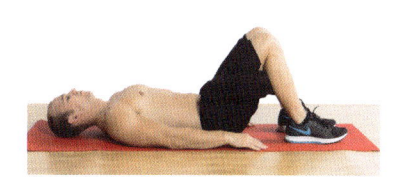

- Begin with both feet on the floor.

NOTES

- Make sure to maintain a stable lumbar spine throughout.

Leg Raise

EQUIPMENT: None

PRIME MOVER: Psoas major

ASSISTANT MOVER: Iliacus

STABILIZERS: Rectus abdominis, internal and external obliques, transverse abdominis

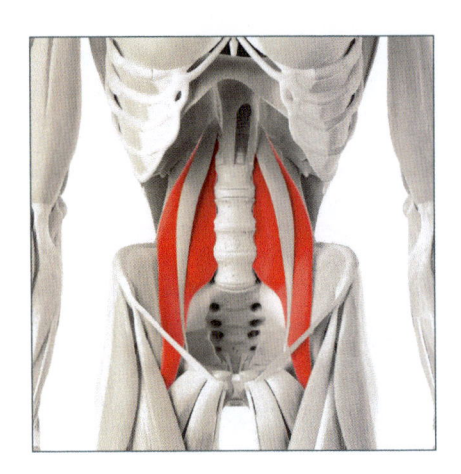

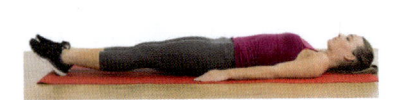

1. Lie face-up with your arms by your sides and your legs fully extended.

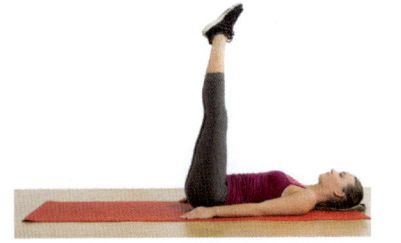

2. Making sure not to overarch your back throughout the movement, brace your abdominals and lift your legs from your hips. At the top of the movement, your feet should be pointing toward the ceiling with your legs straight.

Slowly lower back to the starting position.

Dumbbell Leg Lift

EQUIPMENT: Dumbbell

PRIME MOVERS: Hip flexor muscles

STABILIZERS: Core muscles

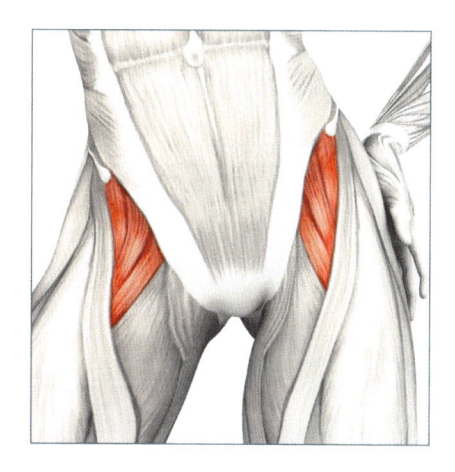

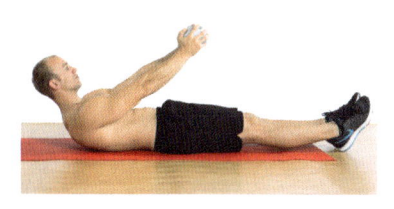

1. Lie face-up with your legs fully extended and your heels on the floor. Curl your trunk up, with a dumbbell in your hands and your arms extended in front of you.

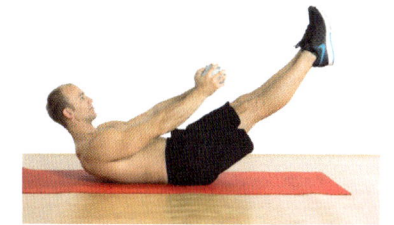

2. Maintaining the trunk position, brace your core and lift your legs. At the top of the movement, your knees should remain straight and your shins should be within a couple inches of touching your hands.

Slowly lower back to the starting position.

NOTES

- Movement should only occur at the hips.

QUADRICEPS

The quadriceps are responsible for extension at the knee and consist of four muscles.

Muscles & Actions

Rectus femoris: This extends the knee as well as assists in flexion at the hip.

Vastus medialis: This assists with extension at the knee as well as patellar stabilization.

Vastus intermedius: This assists with extension at the knee.

Lastus lateralus: This assists with extension at the knee.

Training Tips

- When performing exercises for the quadriceps, leg and foot positioning are important for both safety as well as effectiveness. Pay close attention to the positioning notes.

- Quadriceps exercises should be performed fluidly and controlled.

Floor Leg Extension

EQUIPMENT: None

PRIME MOVERS: Quadriceps

ASSISTANT MOVERS: Psoas major, gluteal muscles

STABILIZERS: Deltoids, pectoralis, core muscles

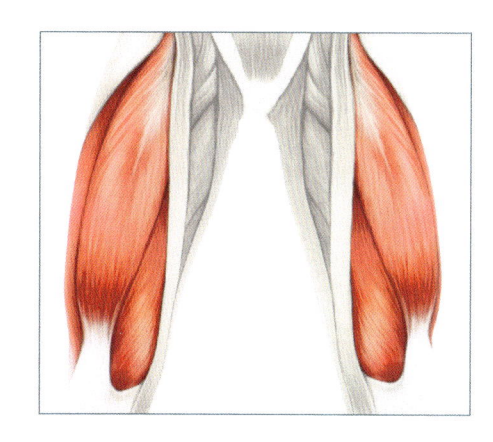

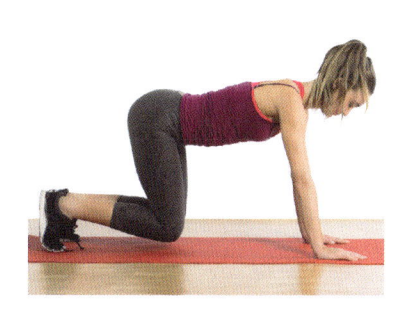

1. Assume a quadruped position and lift your knees off of the floor.

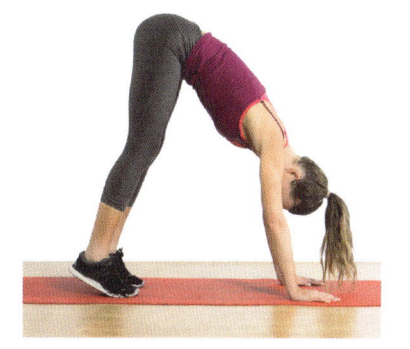

2. Extend your knees, placing yourself in a pike position with your hips higher than your head.

Bend your knees and return to the starting position.

FREEWEIGHT TRAINING ANATOMY

Barbell Squat

EQUIPMENT: **Barbell**

PRIME MOVERS: **Quadriceps**

ASSISTANT MOVERS: **Hamstrings, gluteal muscles**

STABILIZERS: **Erector spinae, rectus abdominis, internal and external obliques**

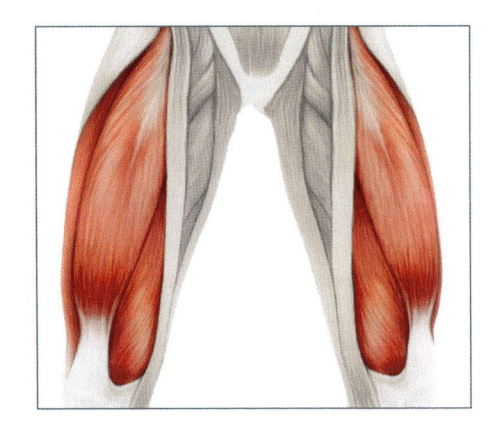

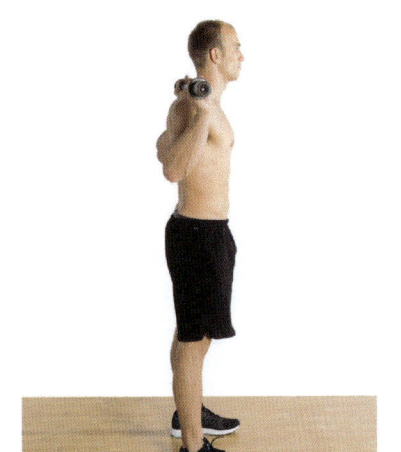

1. Stand with a bar across the upper part of your trapezius (your upper back). Your arms should be bent and lightly holding the bar, securing it in place. Your legs should be between hip- and shoulder-width apart with your toes pointing straight ahead.

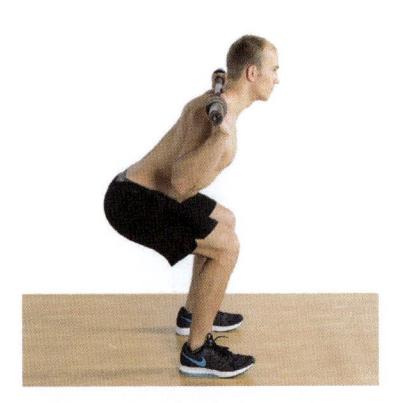

2. Sit back and lower yourself to the floor, bending equally at the knees and the hips. Stop when your thighs are close to parallel to the floor. Your knees should be in line with your toes and your heels should be on the floor.

Drive back up through your heels, engaging your quadriceps and gluteal muscles.

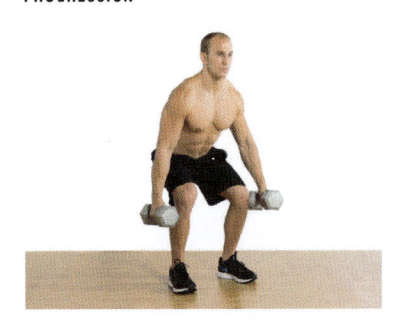

PROGRESSION

- This can also be done with dumbbells. Hold a dumbbell in each hand with your palms facing each other and arms along your sides.

REGRESSION

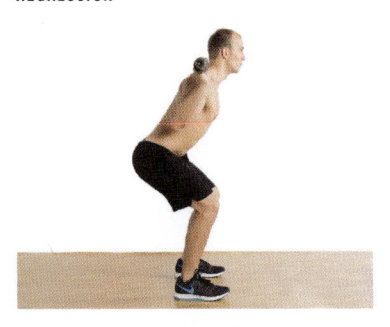

- Lower down only halfway or three-quarters.
- This can also be done with your bodyweight.

NOTES

- Your trunk and calves should be as close to parallel as you can get them.
- Make sure that your knees don't pass in front of your toes.
- Don't overarch your back.

QUADRICEPS

Dumbbell Lunge

EQUIPMENT: Dumbbells

PRIME MOVERS: Quadriceps

ASSISTANT MOVERS: Hamstrings, gluteal muscles

STABILIZERS: Core muscles, deltoids, trapezius, biceps, triceps, forearm muscles

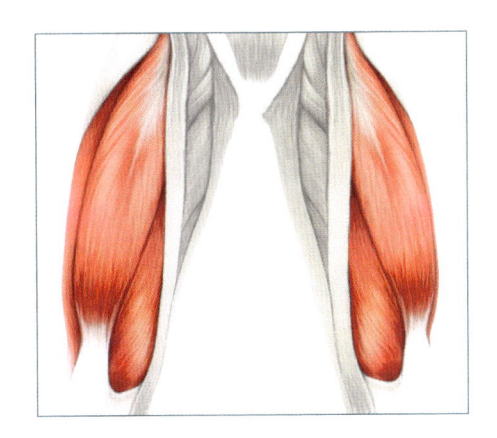

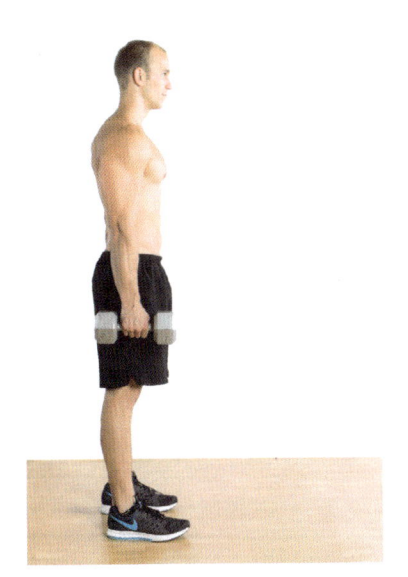

1. Stand upright with a dumbbell in each hand, arms hanging by your sides.

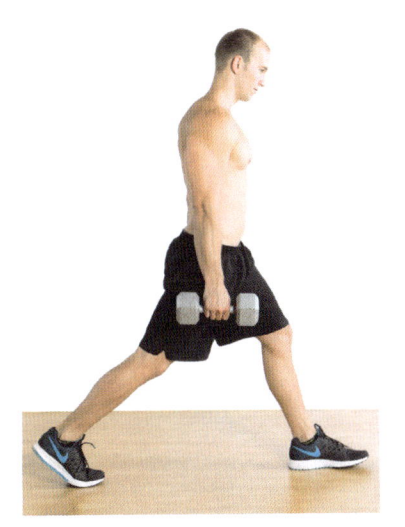

2. Take a step forward and land on your heel. As you step, lift up to the toes of your rear leg.

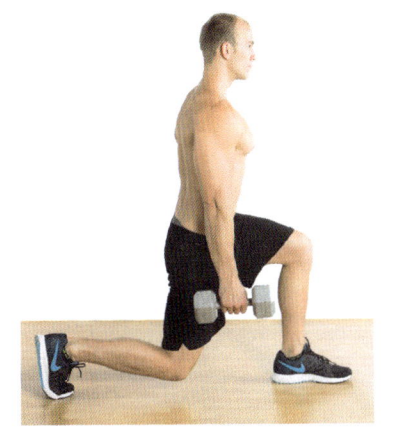

3. Lower straight to the floor by bending both knees until your rear knee is 1 to 3 inches from the floor.

In one motion, drive through your front heel and press back up to the starting position.

Kettlebell Lunge Passthrough

EQUIPMENT: **Kettlebell**

PRIME MOVER: **Quadriceps**

ASSISTANT MOVERS: **Gluteal muscles, hamstrings, deltoids**

STABILIZERS: **Biceps, triceps, forearm muscles**

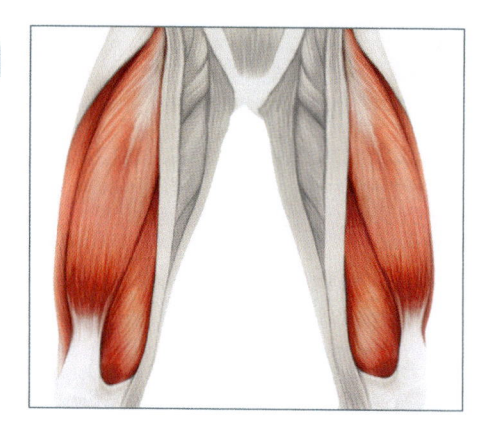

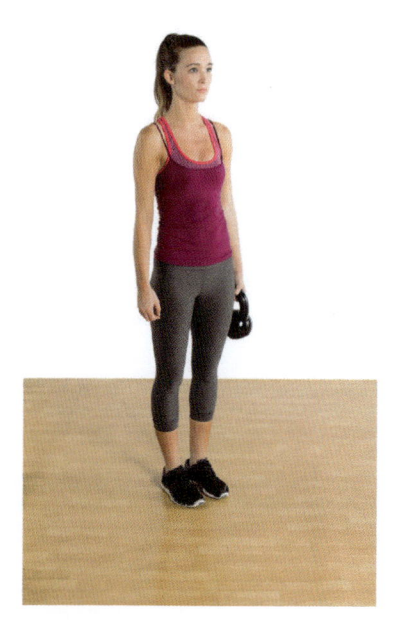

1. Stand upright with a kettlebell in one hand.

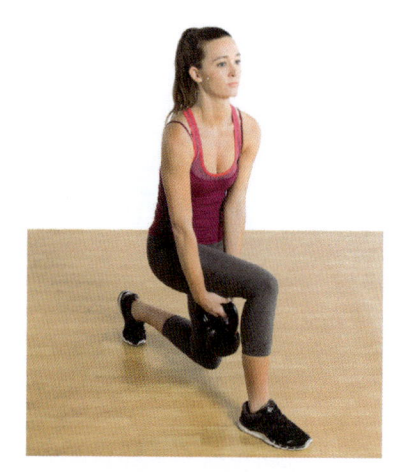

2. Take a step forward and land on your heel. As you step, lift up to the toes of your rear leg. Lower straight to the floor by bending both knees until your rear knee is 1 to 3 inches from the floor. Pass the kettlebell between the legs to your other hand. In one motion, drive through your front heel and press back up to the starting position.

QUADRICEPS 73

Explosive Squat Jump

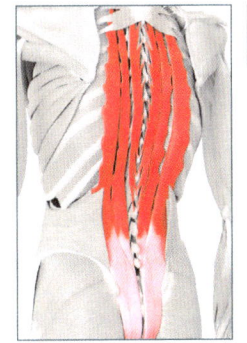

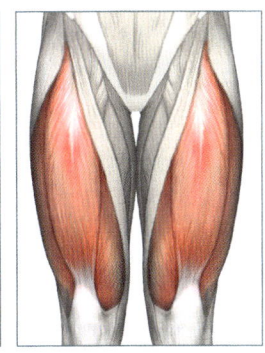

EQUIPMENT: Step, box, or an elevated surface
PRIME MOVERS: Quadriceps, erector spinae
ASSISTANT MOVERS: Calves, gluteal muscles
STABILIZERS: Core muscles, forearm muscles
PREREQUISITE EXERCISE: Barbell squat (page 70)

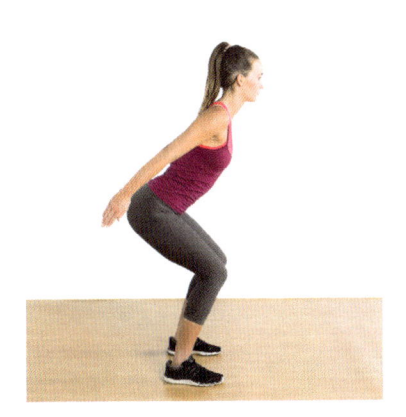

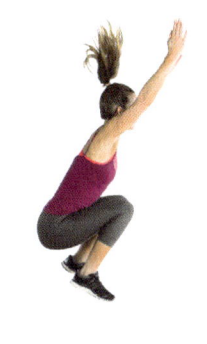

PROGRESSION

- Add a knee tuck at the highest point of your jump.
- Jump onto a stable, elevated surface.

1. Stand upright with your feet hip- to shoulder-width apart and your toes pointing straight ahead. Sit back and lean forward while extending your arms behind you.

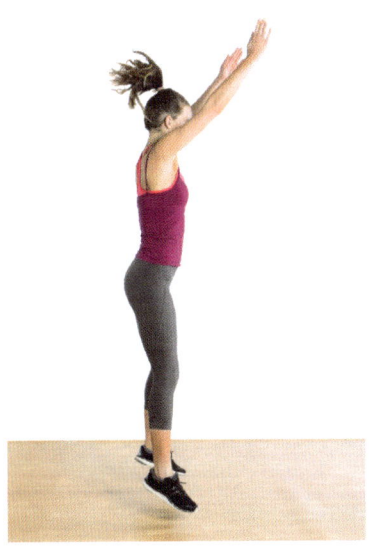

2. Swing your arms up, using the momentum of the arm swing to begin extending your trunk and eventually extending your legs, lifting yourself off of the floor. At the top of the movement, your arms should be fully extended overhead, your trunk should be neutral with a slight extension in the lumbar spine, your knees should be fully extended, and your ankles should be plantarflexed.

As you begin to fall, flex your ankle, knees, and trunk in order to absorb the impact of the landing. When you touch the floor, continue to flex at the ankle, knees, and trunk.

NOTES

- A soft landing is crucial in order to increase efficiency and prevent injuries.
- It's important to perform each repetition as quickly and powerfully as you can.

HAMSTRINGS

The hamstrings are a group of muscles located on the posterior side of the upper leg (femur). They're responsible for flexion at the knee as well as extension at the hip.

Muscles & Actions

Biceps femoris: This is responsible for flexion at the knee, extension at the hip, and external rotation of the leg.

Semimembranosus: This is responsible for flexion at the knee, extension at the hip, and internal rotation of the leg.

Semitendinosus: This is responsible for flexion at the knee, extension at the hip, and internal rotation of the leg.

Training Tips

- The hamstrings are often tight so make sure to properly warm up prior to exercise.
- Make sure to stretch the hamstrings after exercise.
- Perform exercises through a complete ROM in order to avoid exacerbating any preexisting tightness.

Physioball Hamstring Curl

EQUIPMENT: Physioball
PRIME MOVERS: Hamstrings
ASSISTANT MOVERS: Gluteal muscles
STABILIZERS: Core muscles

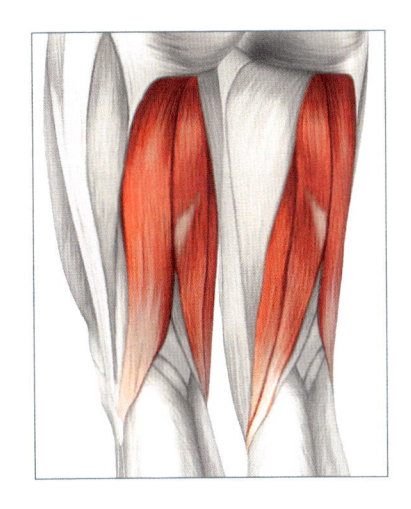

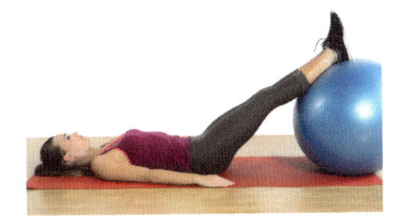

1. Lie face-up on the floor with your legs fully extended, your heels on top of a physioball, and your arms along your sides.

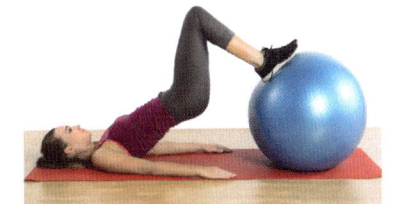

2. Lift your hips off of the floor into a bridge. Bend your knees and curl the ball in as far as you comfortably can.

Lower back to the starting position.

Straight-Leg Deadlift

EQUIPMENT: **Barbell**

PRIME MOVERS: **Hamstrings**

ASSISTANT MOVERS: **Gluteus maximus, erector spinae**

STABILIZERS: **Core muscles, gluteus medius, biceps, triceps, upper back muscles**

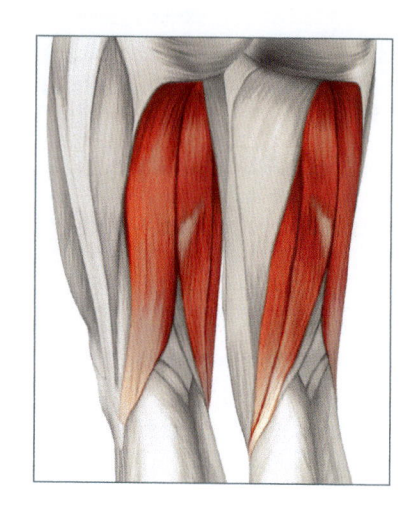

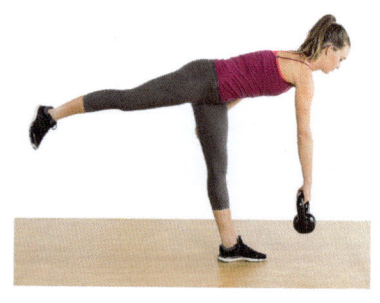

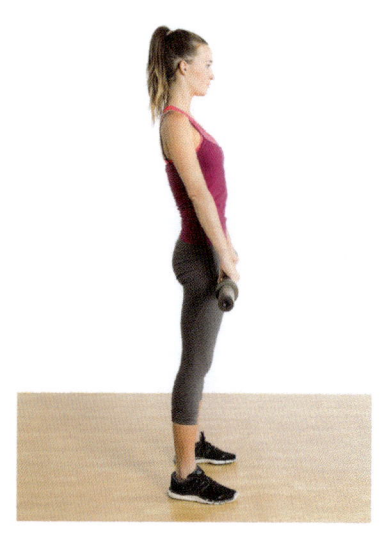

PROGRESSION

1. Stand upright and hold a bar in front of you with your palms facing down, hands shoulder-width apart, and arms straight.

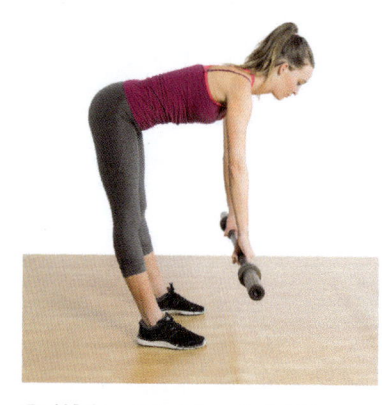

2. While maintaining straight legs, lower your torso from the hips as low as you comfortably can while maintaining a neutral spine.

Extend back up to the starting position.

- Stand upright with a kettlebell in your right hand. Lift your right foot off of the floor and extend the leg behind you.

- While keeping your knee extended and your free leg straight and in line with your torso, lower from your hips as low as you comfortably can while maintaining a neutral spine. Your arms should be hanging while holding the kettlebell.

NOTES

- Make sure to maintain a neutral spine throughout.

Nordic Hamstring Curl

EQUIPMENT: None

PRIME MOVERS: Hamstrings

ASSISTANT MOVER: Gastrocnemius

STABILIZERS: Soleus, core muscles, hip flexors

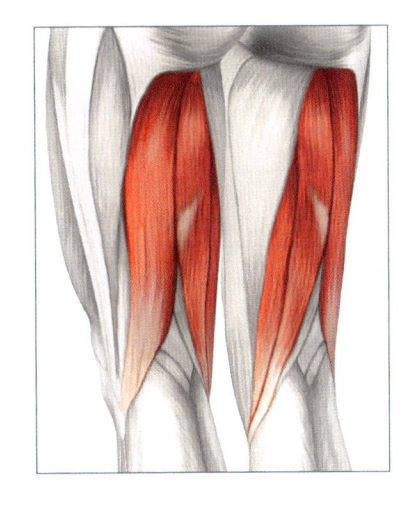

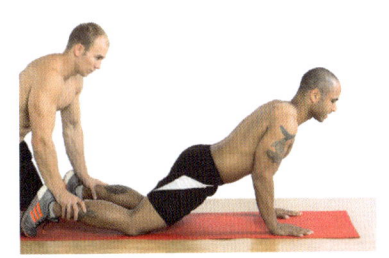

REGRESSION

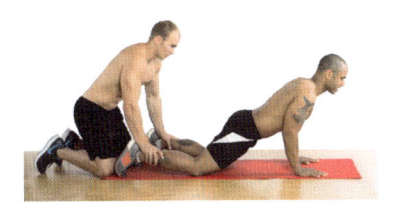

1. Kneel upright. Your legs will need to be fixed in place, either by a partner or a solid structure. Your arms should be bent and at your sides with your hands near your chest.

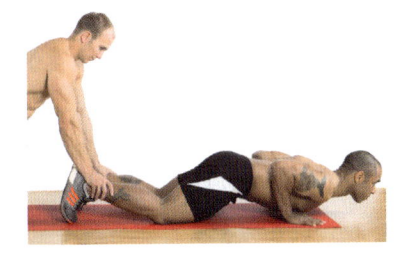

2. Slowly lower yourself by extending your knees. As you reach the floor, use your hands to support and control the landing. Make sure to minimize arm involvement in the exercise. At the bottom of the movement, you should be facedown on the floor with your legs fully extended.

Flex your knees and lift yourself back up to the starting position.

- Use your arms to assist yourself back up.

NOTES

- Maintain a stable spine throughout the movement.

CALF MUSCLES

The calves are a pair of muscles located on the lower leg (tibia and fibula). They're primarily responsible for plantarflexion at the ankle.

Muscles & Actions

Gastrocnemius: This is responsible for plantarflexion of the ankle and assists in flexion at the knee.

Soleus: This assists in plantarflexion at the ankle.

Training Tips

- Since the gastrocnemius acts on two joints, calf exercises with straight legs are the most effective to target them. Alternatively, calf exercises with the knees bent target the soleus.

- The calves are typically very tight so it's important to stretch them, especially after exercise, and avoid overuse.

CALF MUSCLES

Toe Raise

EQUIPMENT: None

PRIME MOVERS: Calves

STABILIZERS: Quadriceps, hamstrings, gluteal muscles

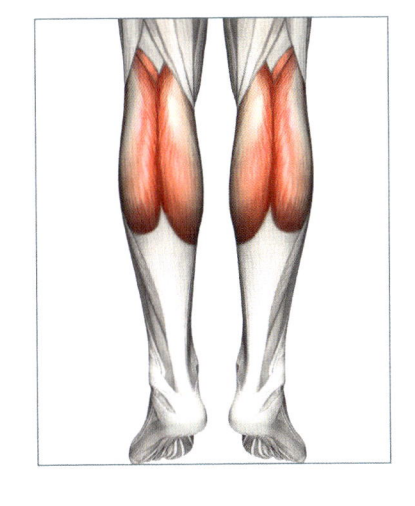

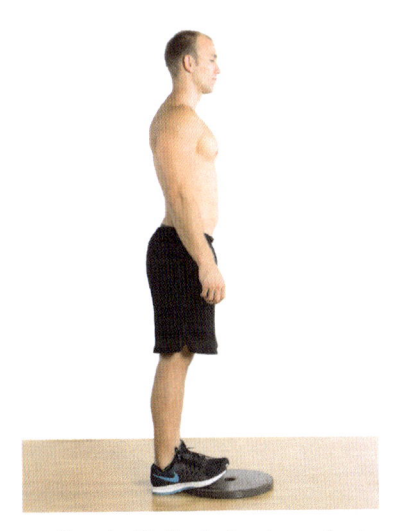

PROGRESSION

1. Stand with the balls of your feet on an elevated surface and the rest of each foot off of the surface. Dorsiflex slightly at your ankles so that your heels are slightly below the level of the surface.

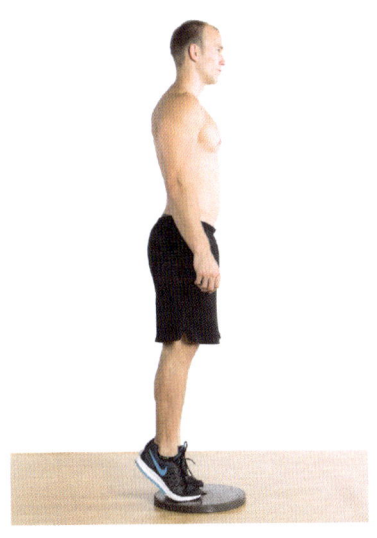

2. Plantarflex your ankles until you're as high as you can comfortably get.

Slowly lower back to the starting position.

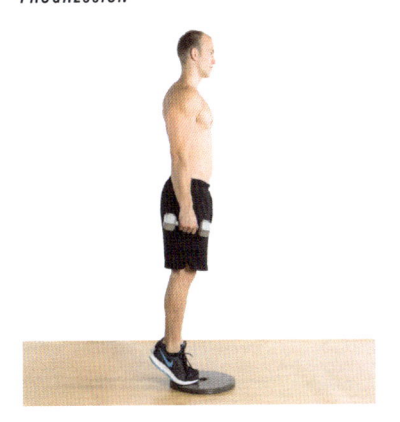

- Hold a weight to add resistance.

REGRESSION

- Perform the exercise on a flat surface.

Seated Calf Raise

EQUIPMENT: **Dumbbell**

PRIME MOVER: **Soleus**

ASSISTANT MOVER: **Gastrocnemius**

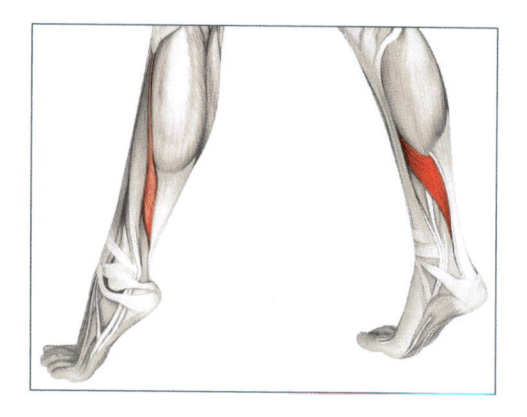

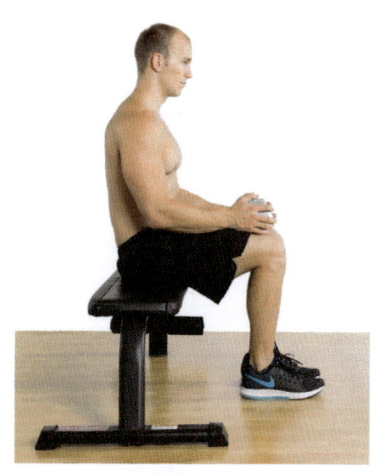

1. Sit with your knees bent and your feet about hip-width apart and flat on the floor. Rest a dumbbell on your thighs.

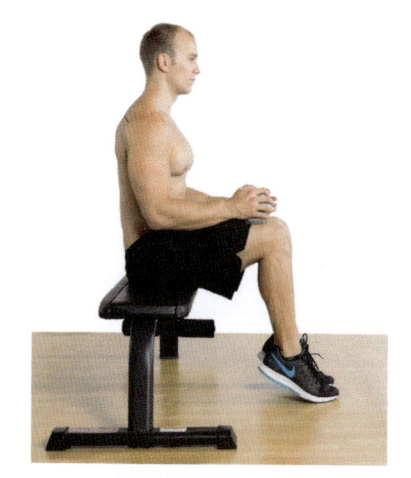

2. Plantarflex your ankles. Lower back to the starting position.

GLUTEAL MUSCLES

The gluteal muscles are a group of muscles located on the backside. They're responsible for extension, abduction, and external rotation at the hips.

Muscles & Actions

Gluteus maximus: This is responsible for extension and external rotation at the hip.

Gluteus medius: This is responsible for abduction as well as internal rotation at the hip.

Gluteus minimus: This is responsible for abduction as well as internal rotation at the hip.

Tensor fasciae latae (TFL): This is responsible for abduction as well as flexion at the hip.

Training Tips

- Often, the muscles of the lower back as well as the hamstrings are involved in exercises focused on the gluteal muscles. In order to maintain focus on the gluteal muscles, be mindful of your positioning.
- Engage your core during gluteal exercises.
- The simple act of thinking of "squeezing your glutes" can be an effective way to increase gluteal activation.

Quadruped Kickback

EQUIPMENT: None

PRIME MOVER: Gluteus maximus

ASSISTANT MOVERS: Erector spinae, hamstrings

STABILIZERS: Core muscles, multifidus

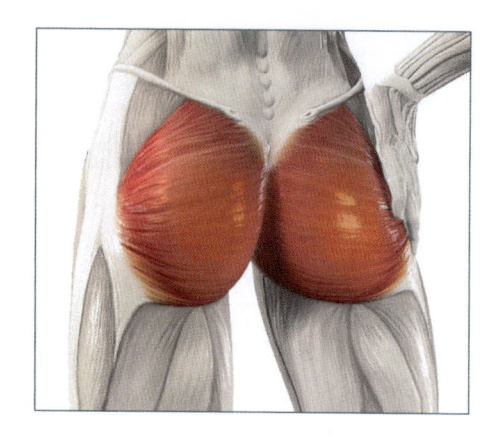

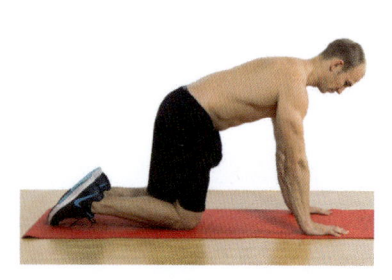

1. Begin in a quadruped position.

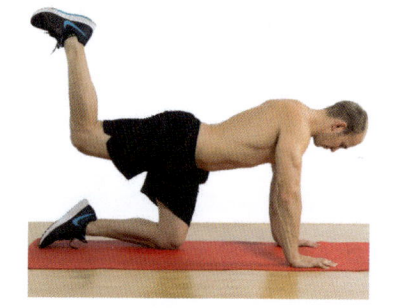

2. Maintaining the bend in your knee, extend one leg from your hip until your upper thigh is slightly above parallel to the floor.

Lower back to the starting position.

GLUTEAL MUSCLES 83

Side-Lying Abduction

EQUIPMENT: None
PRIME MOVERS: Gluteus medius, gluteus minimus
ASSISTANT MOVERS: Sartorius, tensor fasciae latae
STABILIZERS: Piriformis, core muscles

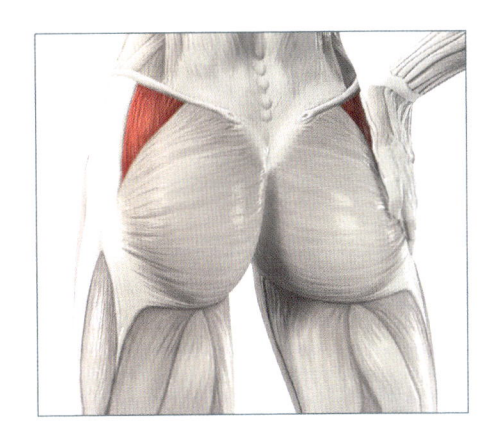

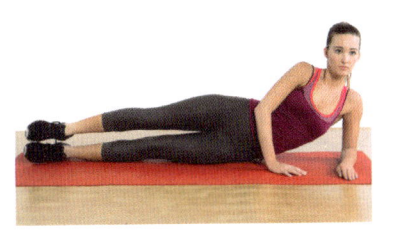

1. Lie on your side.

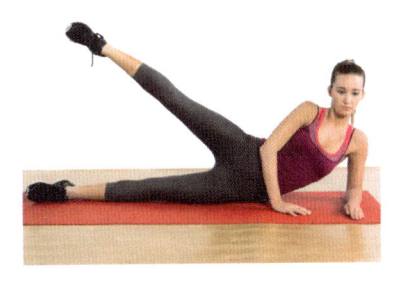

2. Raise your top leg as high as you comfortably can; avoid rotating your hip as you perform the movement.

Lower back to the starting position.

Single-Leg Bridge

EQUIPMENT: None
PRIME MOVER: Gluteus maximus
ASSISTANT MOVERS: Hamstrings
STABILIZERS: Core muscles

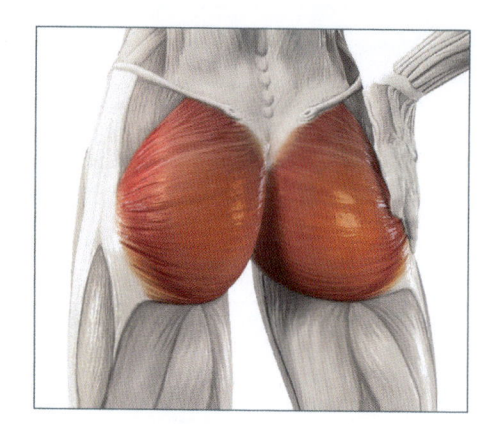

REGRESSION

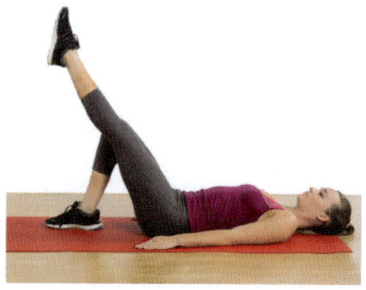

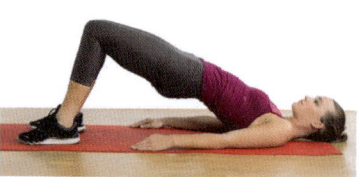

- Perform the movement with both legs on the floor.

1. Lie face-up with your knees bent and your feet on the floor. Lift one leg off of the floor.

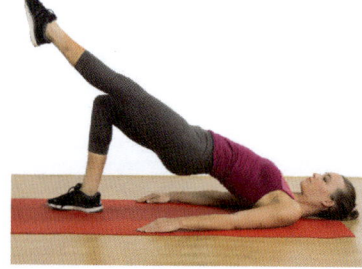

2. Maintaining a neutral lumbar spine throughout the movement, drive up through the planted heel and lift your hips off of the floor as high as you comfortably can.

Lower yourself back to the starting position.

OTHER MUSCLES

This section covers muscles and muscle groups that don't get as much attention as the ones listed earlier. Most of these groups work to assist other, larger muscle groups.

Forearm Muscles

The forearm is located between the elbow and the wrist and consists of muscles that act on the radius and the ulna to maneuver the elbow, wrist, hand, and radioulnar joint. The forearms are very important to exercise as they work during any movement that involves gripping an object. Often, the forearm muscles contract isometrically to hold a weight. Strong forearms are essential to strength training but, since the forearms are constantly working during strength training, it's often not necessary to isolate them for work.

The forearm muscles break down to produce the following movements:

Wrist Extensors

- Extensor carpi ulnaris
- Extensor carpi radialis brevis
- Extensor carpi radialis longus

Wrist Flexors

- Palmaris longus
- Flexor carpi ulnaris
- Flexor carpi radialis

Finger Extensors

- Extensor digitorum
- Extensor indicis
- Extensor pollicis longus
- Extensor pollicis brevis

Finger Flexors

- Flexor digitorum profundus
- Flexor digitorum superficialis
- Flexor pollicis longus

Elbow Extensor

- Anconeus

Pronation

- Pronator teres

Supination

- Supinator

Wrist Curl

EQUIPMENT: **Dumbbell**

PRIME MOVERS: **Wrist flexors**

STABILIZERS: **Biceps, triceps, pronator teres, supinator**

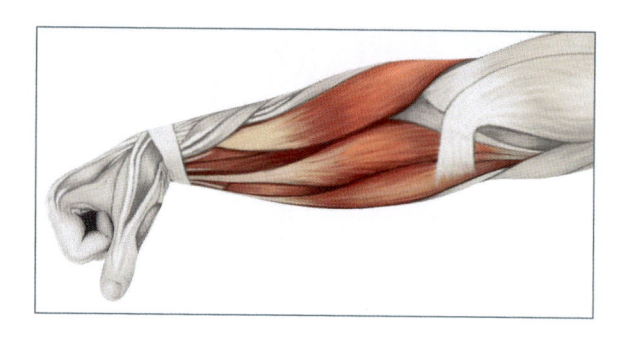

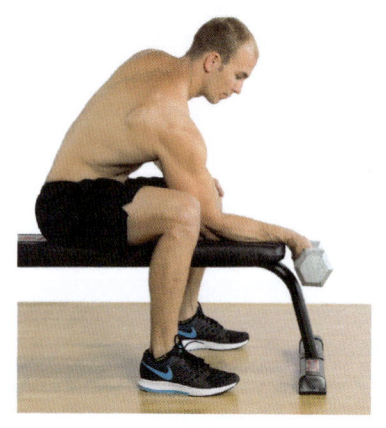

1. Sit with your legs straddling a bench and holding a dumbbell in one hand. Lean forward with a straight back and place one forearm flat on the bench. Your palm should face up and your hand should hang off of the edge of the bench. Extend your wrist as far as you comfortably can.

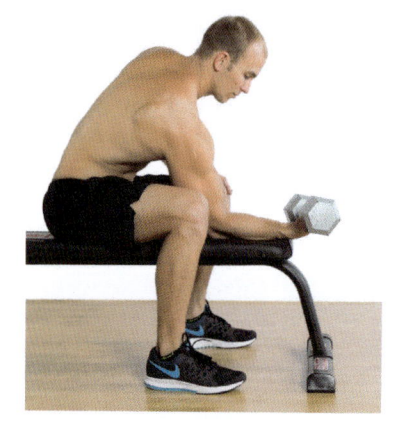

2. Flex your wrist as high as you comfortably can.

Extend back to the starting position.

OTHER MUSCLES 87

Wrist Extension

EQUIPMENT: Dumbbell

PRIME MOVERS: Wrist extensors

STABILIZERS: Biceps, triceps, pronator teres, supinator

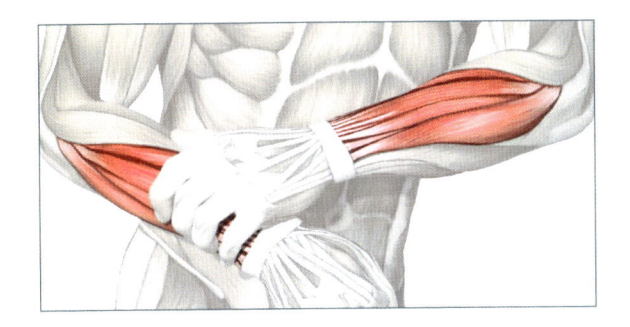

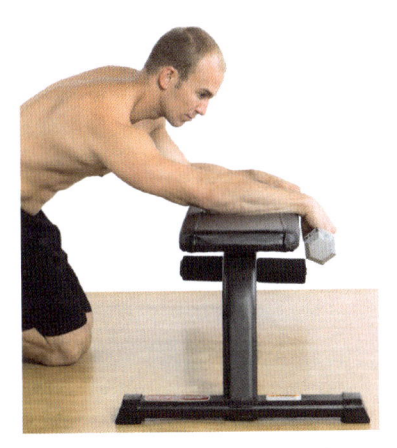

1. Kneel on the floor in front of a bench. While holding a dumbbell palms down in one hand, place your forearm flat on the bench. Your hand should hang off of the edge of the bench. Allow your wrist to curl down to the floor.

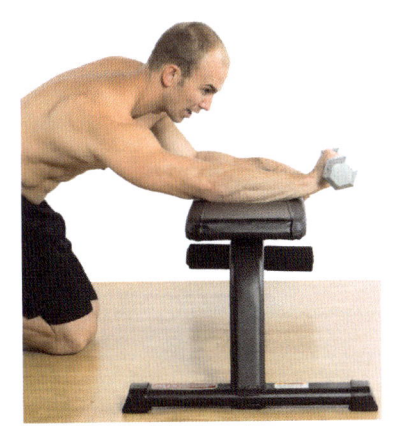

2. Extend your wrist as high as you comfortably can.

Curl back to the starting position.

Pronation/Supination

EQUIPMENT: **Dumbbell**

PRIME MOVERS: **Pronator teres, supinator, biceps brachii**

STABILIZERS: **Wrist flexors, wrist extensors**

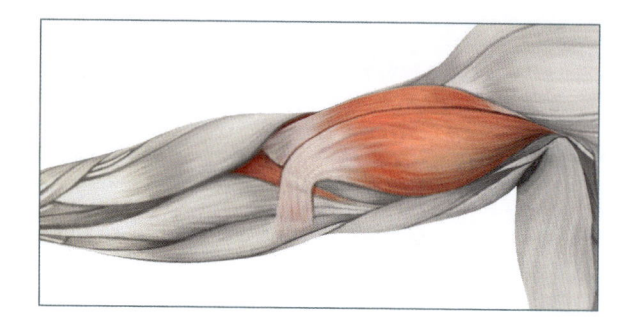

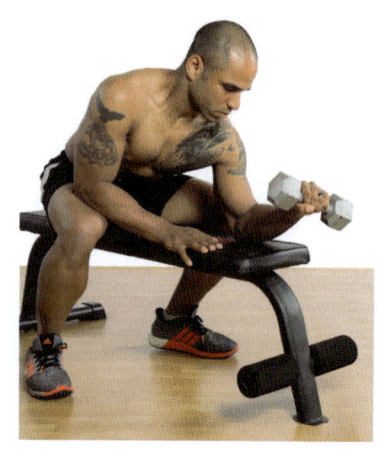

1. Sit with your legs straddling a bench. While holding a dumbbell in one hand, lean forward with a straight back and place one forearm flat on the bench. Your wrist should be in a neutral position with your palm facing down. Keeping your elbow on the bench, elevate your forearm so that the only point with contact is the elbow.

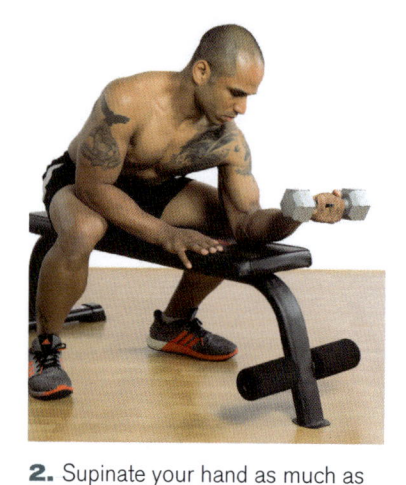

2. Supinate your hand as much as you comfortably can.

Pronate back to the starting position.

> **NOTES**
> - If possible, use a weight that is unevenly distributed so that one side is loaded with more weight than the other.

Rotator Cuff Muscles

The rotator cuff represents one of the more important muscle groups in the body. The rotator cuff plays a role in almost all upper-body movements, acting as a stabilizer by compressing the glenohumeral joint. Additionally, the rotator cuff acts as an internal/external rotator of the humerus.

MUSCLES & ACTIONS

Supraspinatus: This abducts the arm.

Infrispinatus: This externally rotates the arm.

Teres major: This externally rotates the arm.

Subscapularis: This internally rotates the arm.

TRAINING TIPS

- The rotator cuff muscles are both incredibly important and prone to injury. When performing movements for the rotator cuff, follow the instructions precisely.

- These exercises are meant to be used for prehabilitation or rehabilitation purposes and are a great way to prepare the shoulder joint for exercise.

- Technique and ROM should be your primary focus, so use light weights when training the rotator cuff.

- If you experience any pain or discomfort, terminate the exercise immediately.

External Rotation & Press

EQUIPMENT: None

PRIME MOVERS: Infraspinatus, teres major

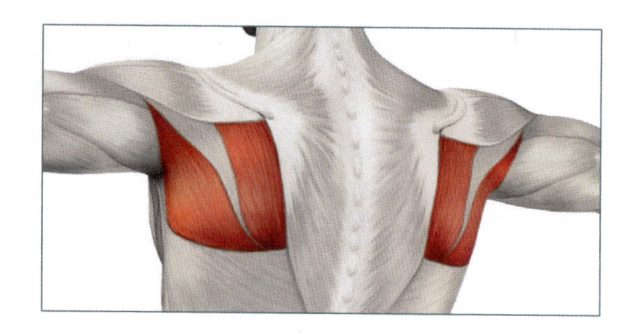

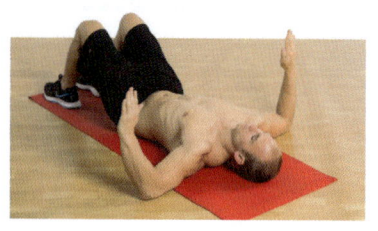

1. Lie face-up with your knees bent. Resting on the ground, your upper arm (humerus) should be abducted and form a "T" with your body. There should be a 90 degree bend in your elbow with your hands pointing up toward the ceiling.

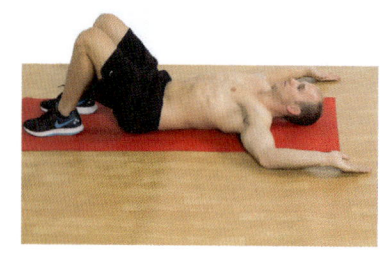

2. Externally rotate your arms and lower your lower arm (radius and ulna) toward the floor. The ROM on this exercise may vary, but lower as far as you comfortably can without pain.

PROGRESSION

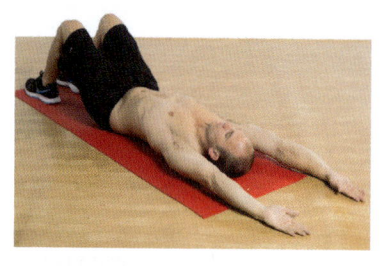

- Extend your arms, sliding your upper arm (humerus) on the floor and alongside your ears.

OTHER MUSCLES 91

External Rotation to Shoulder Press

EQUIPMENT: Dumbbells

PRIME MOVERS: Supraspinatus, teres major, infraspinatus

ASSISTANT MOVERS: Triceps, deltoids

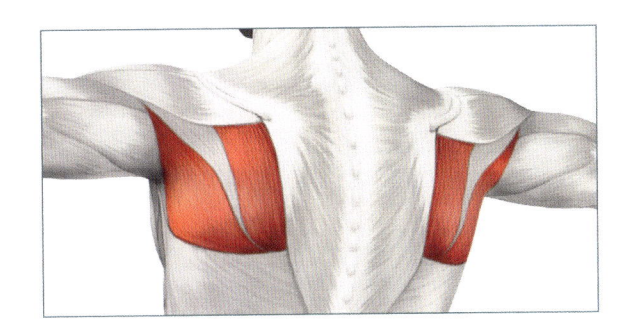

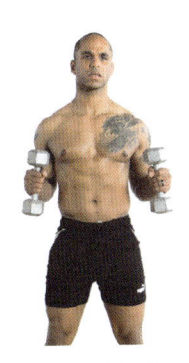

1. Stand upright with your arms by your sides and a dumbbell in each hand. Bend your elbows 90 degrees with your palms facing each other.

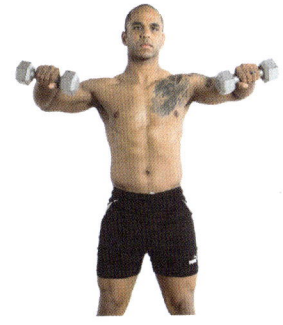

2. Abduct your arms until your upper arms (humerus) are parallel to the floor.

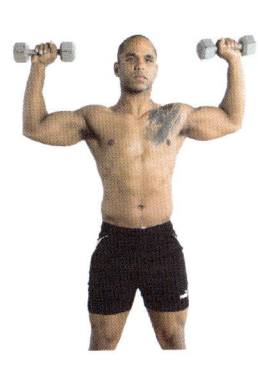

3. Externally rotate your arms until your hands are pointed toward the ceiling.

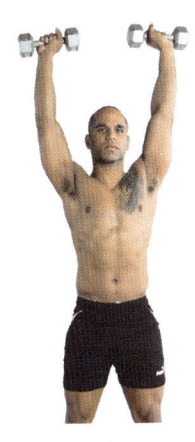

4. Press both arms straight up until your arms are fully extended.

Reverse the movements back to the starting position.

Shin Muscles

The tibial muscles are located on the tibia and fibula (bones of the lower leg) and are responsible for plantarflexion and supination of the foot. The peronei are located on the side of the tibia and fibula and are responsible for plantarflexion and pronation of the foot.

MUSCLES & ACTIONS

Tibialis anterior: This is responsible for dorsiflexion of the foot and assists with supination at the foot.

Tibialis posterior: This is responsible for supination of the foot and assists with plantarflexion.

Peroneus longus: This is responsible for plantarflexion and pronation of the foot.

Peroneus brevis: This is responsible for plantarflexion and pronation of the foot.

Peroneus tertius: This is responsible for dorsiflexion and eversion of the foot.

TRAINING TIPS

- The tibial muscles are typically underemphasized in exercise programming, which contributes to an imbalance that results in tight calves and weak tibial muscles. Tibial exercises should be performed regularly in order to help restore balance between the muscles.

Dorsiflexion & Foot Circle

EQUIPMENT: None

PRIME MOVERS: Tibialis anterior, tibialis posterior, peronei

ASSISTANT MOVERS: Calves

STABILIZERS: Peronei

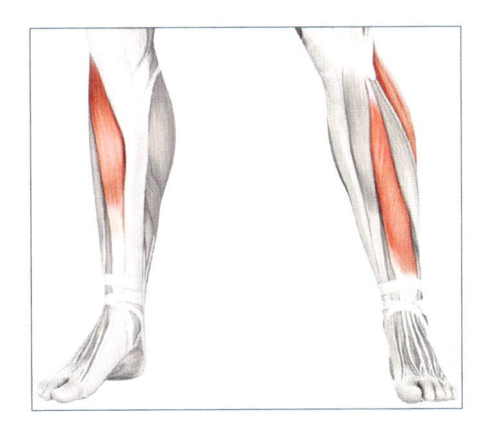

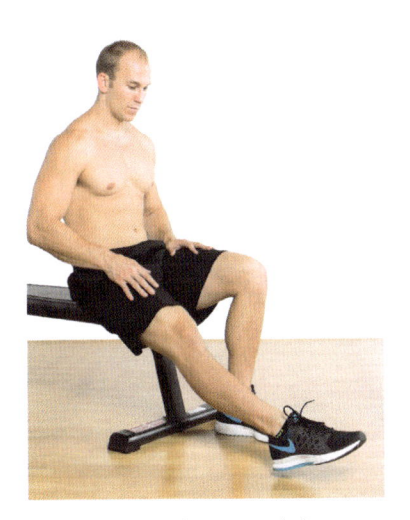

1. Sit with one leg extended so that your foot is off of the floor and plantarflexed.

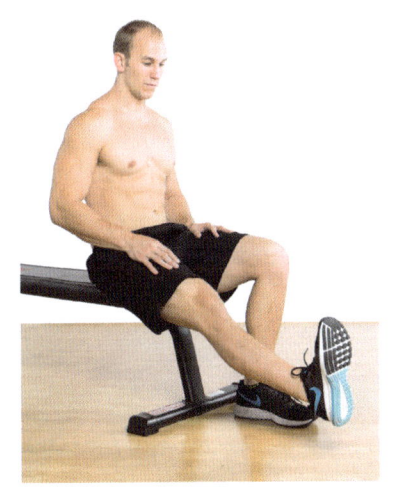

2. Dorsiflex your foot as high as you can.

Plantarflex as far as you can.

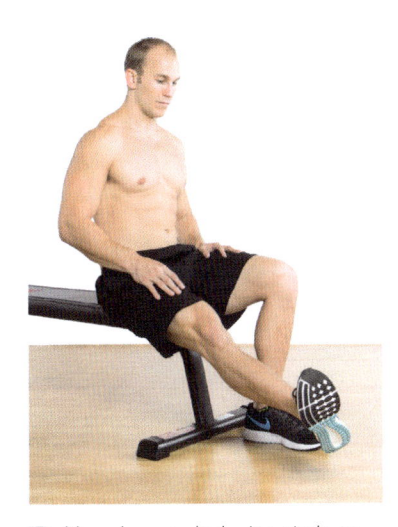

3. Now draw a clockwise circle as large as you can.

After the predetermined number of repetitions, draw counterclockwise circles as large as you can.

Adductor Muscles

The adductor muscles are the muscles responsible for adduction of the thigh.

MUSCLES & ACTIONS

Adductor longus: This is responsible for hip adduction and assists in hip flexion.

Adductor brevis: This is responsible for hip adduction and assists in hip flexion.

Adductor magnus: This is responsible for hip adduction and assists in hip extension.

TRAINING TIPS

- Adductor muscles are often tight so in addition to strengthening exercises, stretching should be emphasized in order to avoid injuries.

Side Lunge

EQUIPMENT: None
PRIME MOVERS: Adductor muscles
ASSISTANT MOVERS: Quadriceps, gluteal muscles
STABILIZERS: Core muscles, calves, tibial muscles

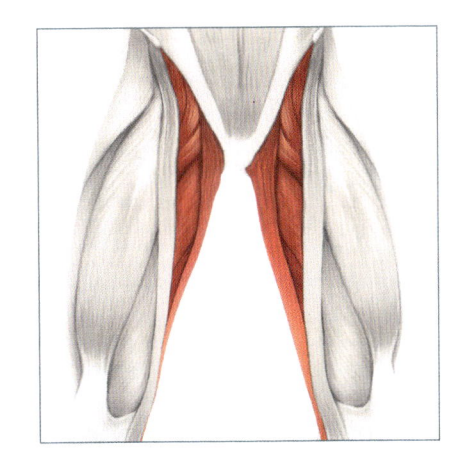

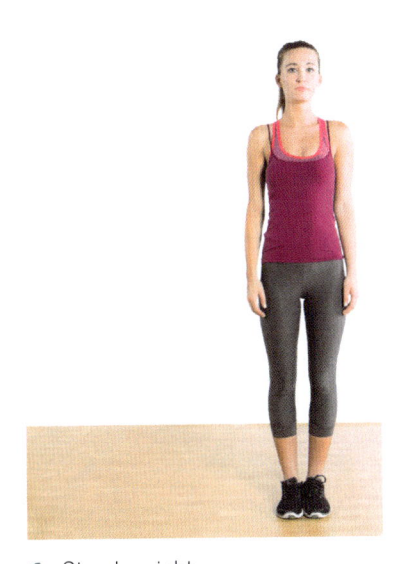

1. Stand upright.

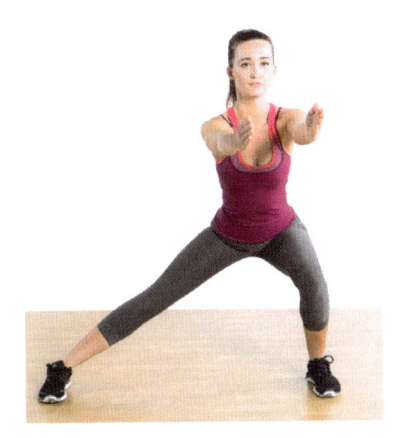

2. While keeping your left leg planted, take a long step to your right. As your foot hits the floor, sit back, lean forward, and extend your arms. At the bottom of the movement, your right leg should be straight with the foot flat on the floor. The left leg and hip should be flexed, and your arms should be extended forward.

Drive through your left heel and press up in one motion to the starting position.

Side Plank with Elevated Bottom Leg

EQUIPMENT: None

PRIME MOVERS: Adductor muscles

STABILIZERS: Obliques, deltoids, rotator cuff

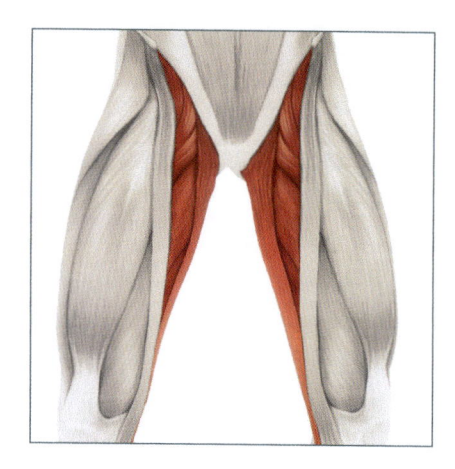

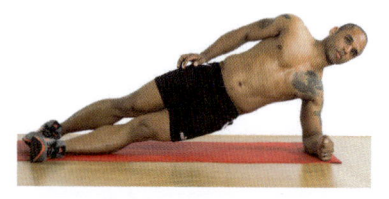

1. Begin in a side plank position with your feet staggered on the floor. Your bottom leg should be in front of the top leg.

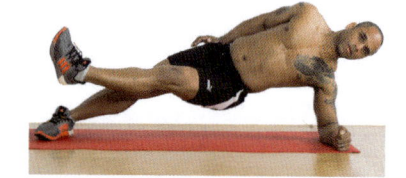

2. Raise your bottom leg as high as you comfortably can.

Lower back to the starting position.

FULL-BODY MOVEMENTS

Full-body movements are exercises that use some combination of upper-body, lower-body, and core muscles to produce movements. They're very effective and necessary as they use the whole body as a unit to produce a movement. Since many of the exercises in this section will reference previous exercises, you may need to look at earlier exercises in this book. In these situations, the page number will be provided.

Squat, Curl, & Press

EQUIPMENT: Dumbbells

PRIME MOVERS: Quadriceps, biceps, deltoids

ASSISTANT MOVERS: Gluteal muscles, triceps

STABILIZERS: Upper back, core muscles, rotator cuff, forearm muscles

PREREQUISITE EXERCISES: Dumbbell squat (page 70), dumbbell biceps curl (page 41), shoulder press (page 35)

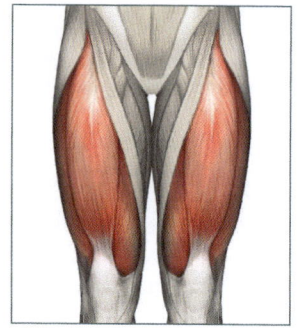

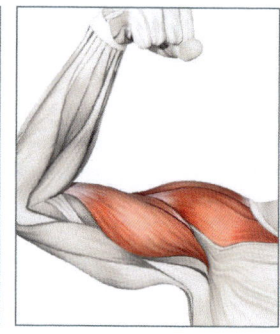

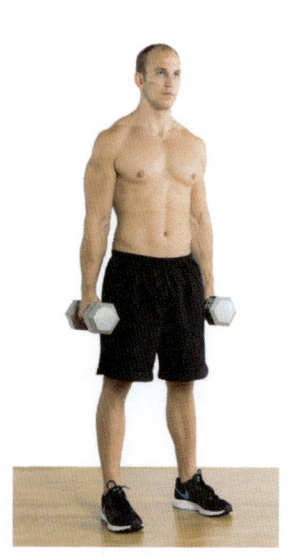

1. Stand upright with your feet between hip- and shoulder-width apart and toes pointing straight ahead. Hold a dumbbell in each hand with your palms facing each other and arms along your sides.

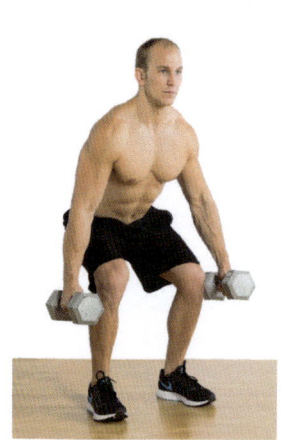

2. Lower into a squat.

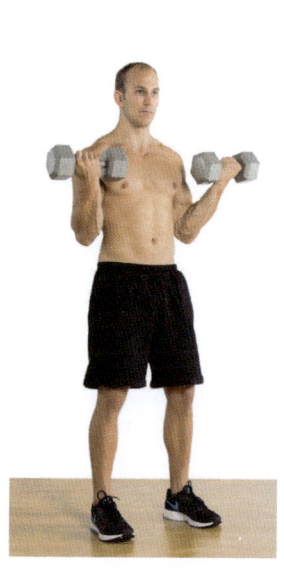

3. Now straighten your legs and, at the same time, bend your elbows to bring the dumbbells toward your shoulders.

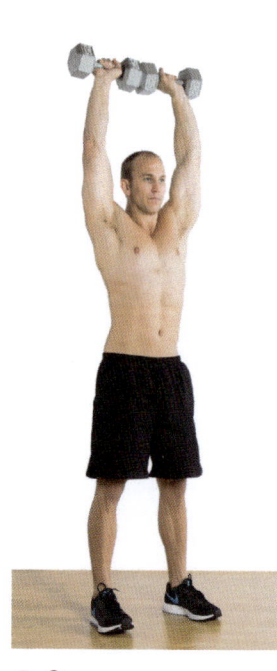

4. Once your arms are fully flexed, simultaneously turn your palms away from you while pressing the dumbbells up to the ceiling.

Return back to the starting position.

Side Lunge with Sword Draw

EQUIPMENT: Dumbbell

PRIME MOVERS: Deltoids, adductors

ASSISTANT MOVERS: Rotator cuff, upper back muscles, quadriceps, gluteal muscles

STABILIZERS: Core muscles, calves, forearm muscles

PREREQUISITE EXERCISES: Side lunge (page 95)

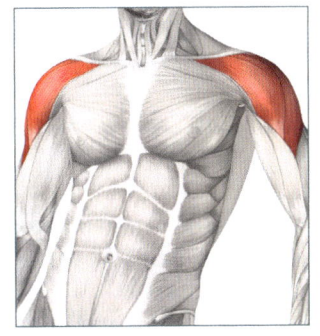

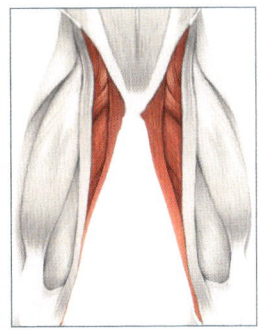

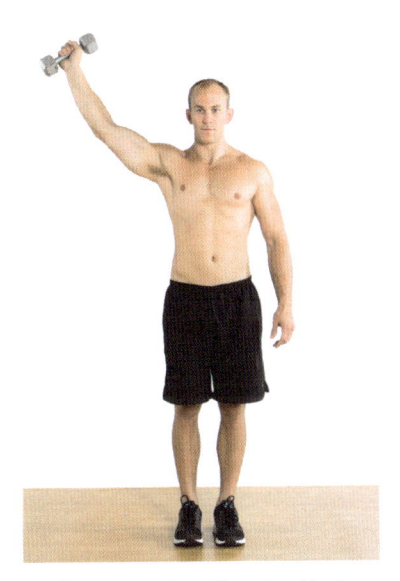

1. Stand upright with a dumbbell in your right hand. Your right arm should be straight and extended diagonally about 45 degrees.

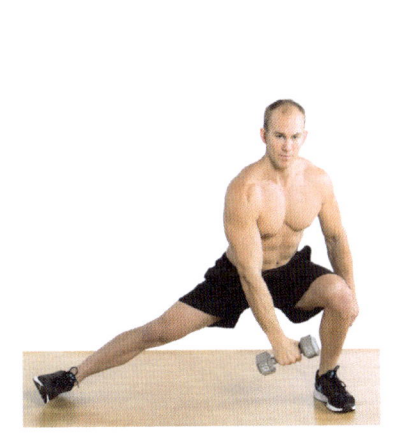

2. Take a long step to your left. As your foot hits the floor, sit back, lean forward, and reach across your body with your right arm.

At the bottom of the movement, your right leg should be straight and your left leg flexed with your thigh parallel to the floor. Your torso should be bent at the waist with a straight back and your arm should be straight and reaching across your body.

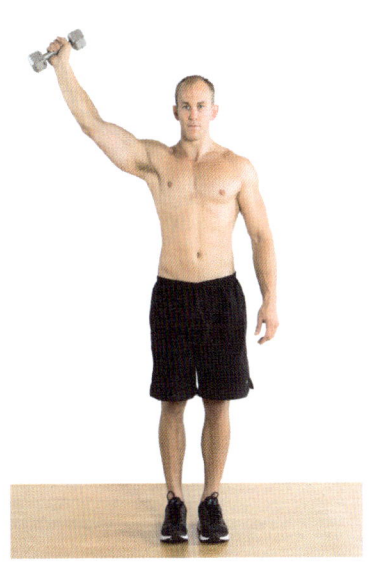

3. In one motion, drive through your right heel back to the starting leg position while simultaneously extending your arm diagonally from the shoulder.

Sandbag Lunge & Rotation

EQUIPMENT: Sandbag

PRIME MOVERS: Quadriceps, internal and external obliques

ASSISTANT MOVERS: Gluteal muscles, hamstrings

STABILIZERS: Biceps, triceps, deltoids, forearm muscles

PREREQUISITE EXERCISES: Dumbbell lunge (page 71)

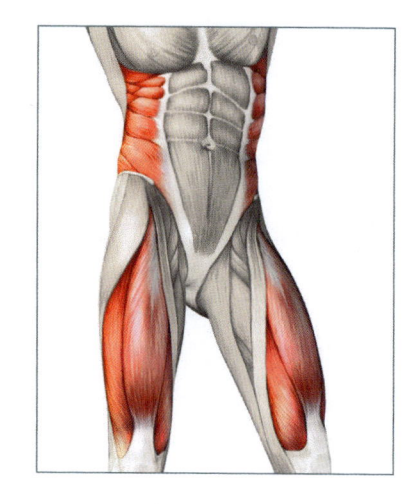

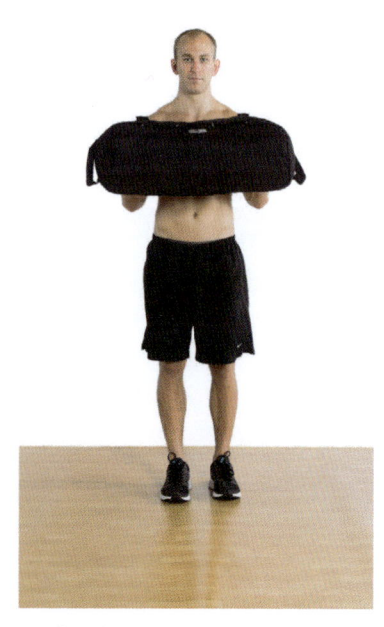

1. Stand and hold a sandbag at chest level.

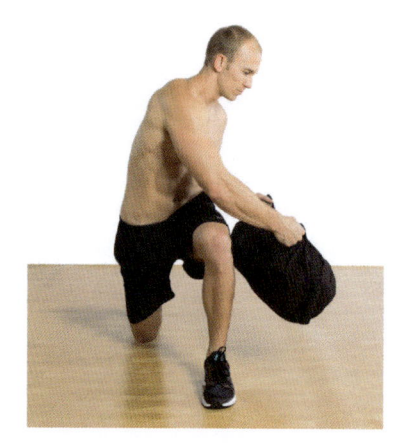

2. Step forward and lunge with your left leg. As your foot hits the floor, lower the sandbag and rotate to your left side. At the bottom of the movement, you should be in a full lunge and rotated to your left. Your arms should be fully extended and holding the sandbag on the outside of your left leg.

Drive back up to the starting position.

Deadlift

EQUIPMENT: Barbell
PRIME MOVERS: Latissimus dorsi, upper back muscles, quadriceps
ASSISTANT MOVERS: Hamstrings, gluteal muscles
STABILIZERS: Core muscles, biceps, triceps, deltoids, forearm muscles
PREREQUISITE EXERCISE: Barbell squat (page 70)

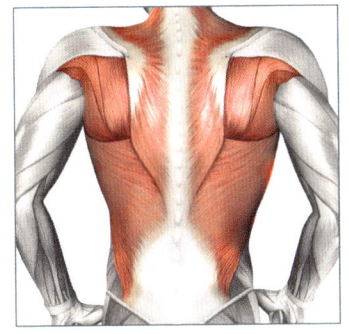

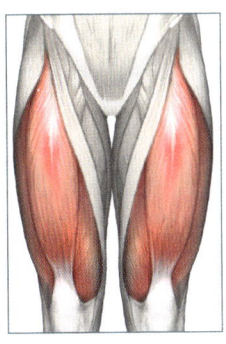

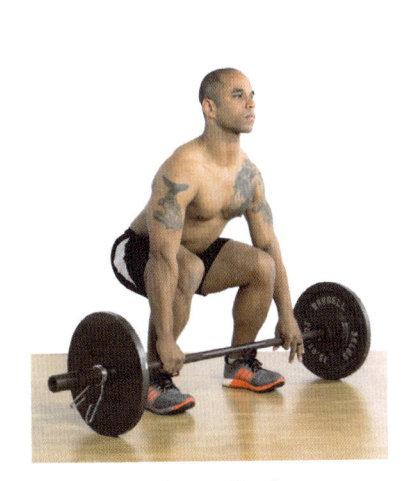

1. Place the bar on the floor or an elevated surface. Stand behind the bar with your feet between hip- and shoulder-width apart. Sit back into a squat and grip the bar with your hands slightly wider than your legs.

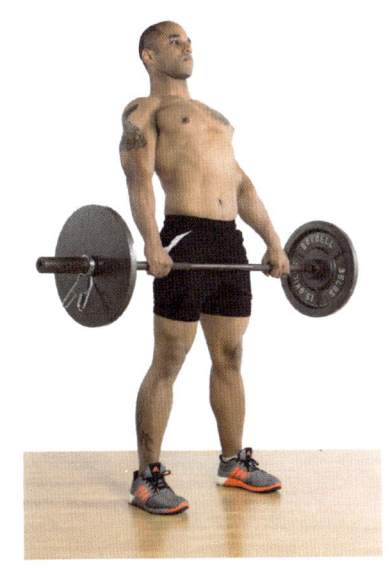

2. Drive through your heels and extend your legs and torso up to standing.

Sit back into a squat and lower the bar back to the floor.

Kettlebell Renegade Row

EQUIPMENT: **Kettlebells**

PRIME MOVERS: **Pectoralis major, latissimus dorsi**

ASSISTANT MOVER: **Biceps**

STABILIZERS: **Core muscles, quadriceps, hamstrings, rotator cuff muscles, biceps, triceps, forearm muscles**

PREREQUISITE EXERCISES: Push-up (page 13), single-leg kettlebell row (page 26)

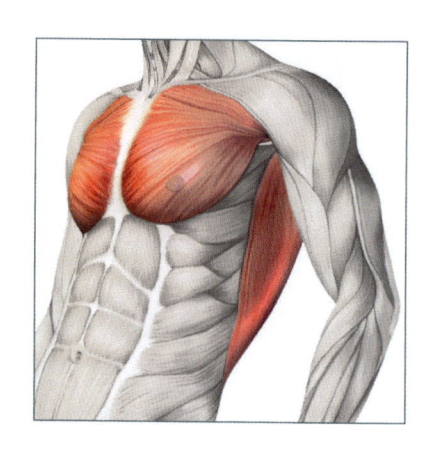

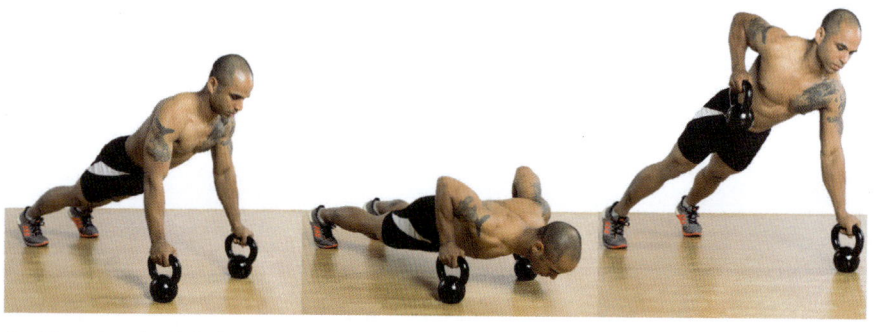

1. Place two kettlebells on the floor and assume the top of a push-up position with each hand gripping the handle of a kettlebell.

2. Lower your chest toward the floor, getting as low as you comfortably can without your chest hitting the floor.

3. Press up to the starting position. As you reach the top, pull one kettlebell up off of the floor as high as you can comfortably can using a rowing motion, keeping your arm close to your torso. At the top of the movement, your torso should remain stable with minimal rotation.

Lower the kettlebell back to the floor.

REGRESSION

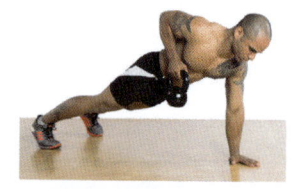

- Perform the same movement with one hand on the floor and one hand on a kettlebell.

FULL-BODY MOVEMENTS 103

Kettlebell Swing

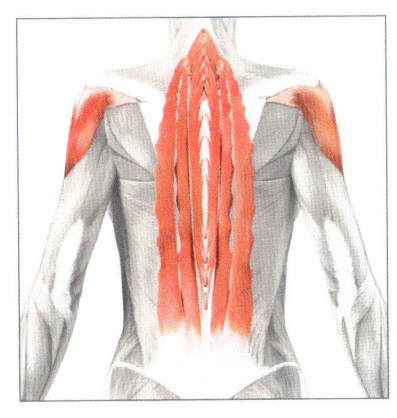

EQUIPMENT: Kettlebell

PRIME MOVERS: Deltoids, erector spinae

ASSISTANT MOVERS: Gluteal muscles, upper back muscles, hamstrings

STABILIZERS: Core muscles, biceps, triceps, forearm muscles

PREREQUISITE EXERCISE: Deadlift (page 101)

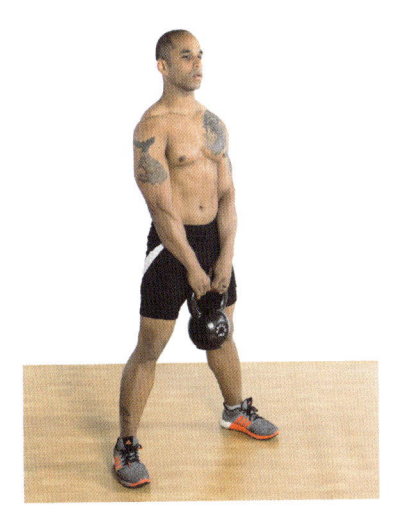

PROGRESSION

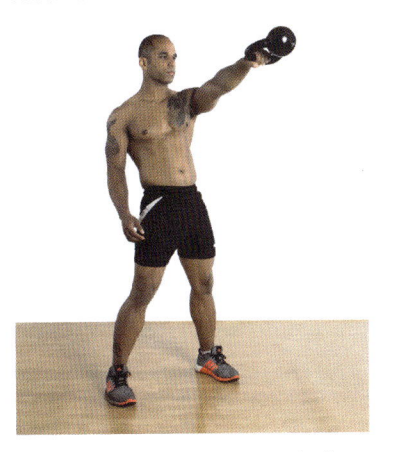

1. Stand upright with your feet shoulder-width apart. With your arms extended down and between your legs, hold a kettlebell with both hands.

NOTES

- Maintain a stable core and neutral spine throughout the movement.
- While your knees will bend, make sure that the movement comes from the hip drive, not squatting.
- Utilize momentum throughout the movement.

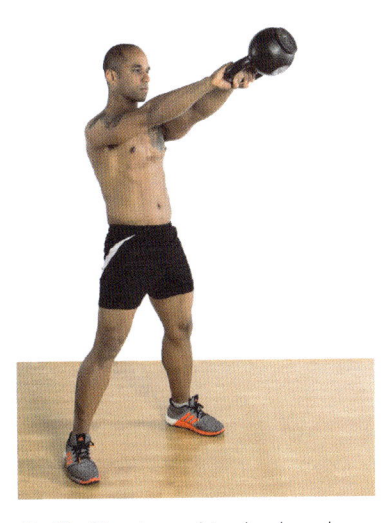

2–3. Shoot your hips back and swing the kettlebell between your legs, then quickly transition and thrust your hips forward, using the momentum to lift your arms until they're fully extended and approximately eye level. Your trunk should be neutral with your core muscles engaged while extending back slightly. Your legs should also be fully extended.

Quickly transition back down while shooting your hips back.

- Do this with one arm instead of two.

Turkish Get-Up

EQUIPMENT: Kettlebell

PRIME MOVERS: Hip flexor muscles, quadriceps, pectoralis

ASSISTANT MOVERS: Gluteal muscles, hamstrings, triceps

STABILIZERS: Biceps, triceps, deltoids, pectoralis, forearm muscles

PREREQUISITE EXERCISES: Dumbbell press (page 15), sit-up (page 52), single-leg bridge (page 84), dumbbell lunge (page 71)

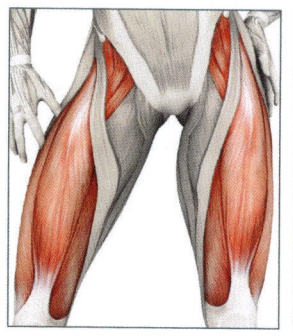

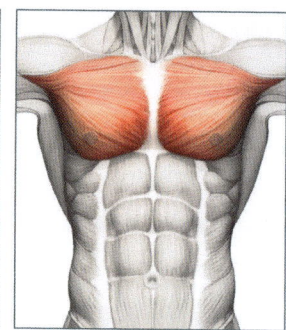

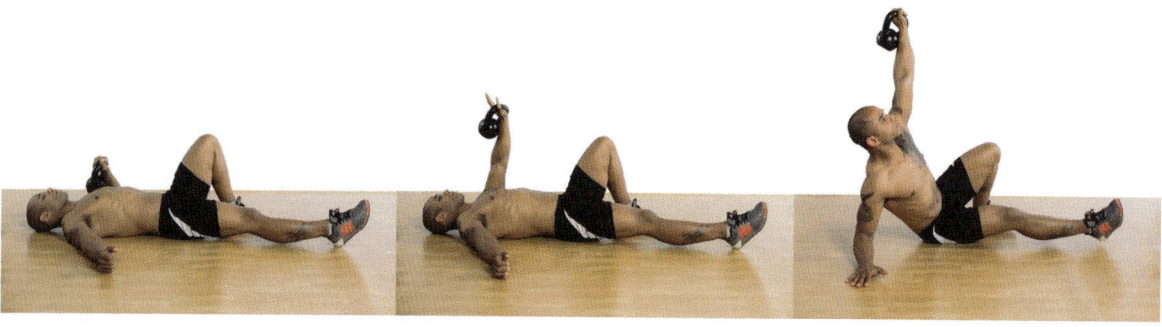

1. Lie face-up with your left leg bent and your foot flat on the floor; your right leg should be fully extended with your heel on the floor. Place your left upper arm flat on the floor by your side and hold a kettlebell in your left hand. Bend your arm 90 degrees with your fist pointing to the ceiling. Your right arm should be extended and abducted about 45 degrees.

2. Press the kettlebell up until your arm is fully extended and pointing up toward the ceiling.

3. Using your right arm for support, sit up while keeping your left hand pointing toward the ceiling.

FULL-BODY MOVEMENTS

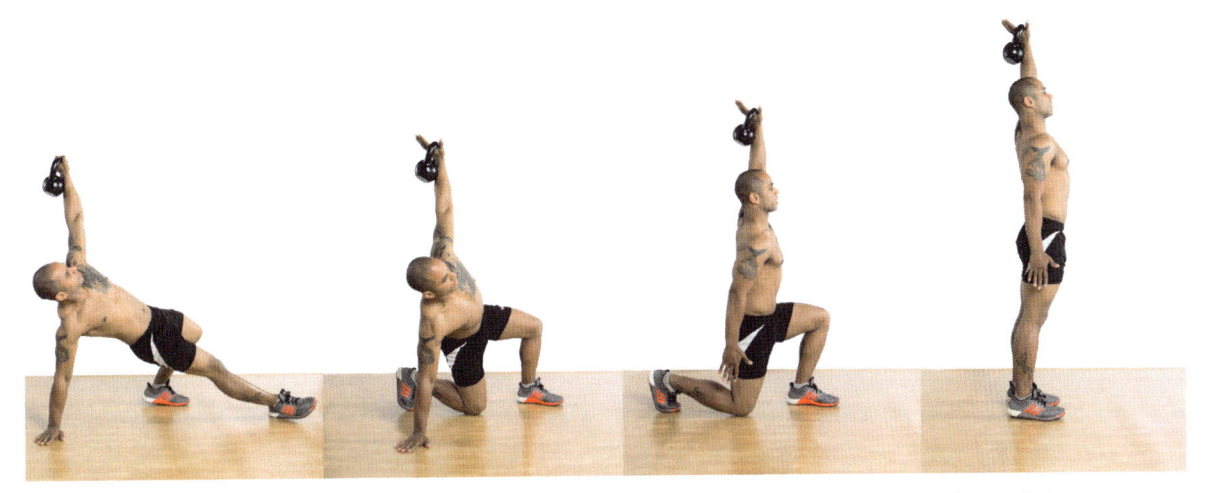

4. Bridge up by lifting your hips off of the floor. At this point, the only points of contact with the floor should be your left foot, your right heel, and your right palm.

5. Pull your right leg all the way behind you and place your right knee on the floor.

6. Straighten out your torso. At this point, both knees should be flexed 90 degrees, with your left foot and right knee on the floor. Your torso should be in a neutral position with your left arm still extended and pointing up toward the ceiling.

7. Stand all the way up so that your feet are together, your torso is upright, and your arm is extended straight up.

Reverse the steps to get back to the starting position.

Kettlebell Anyhow

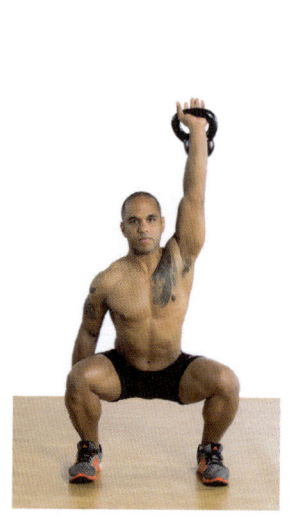

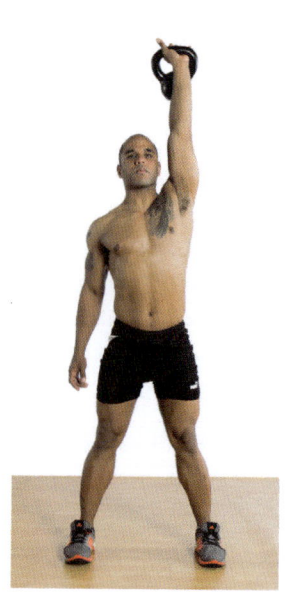

EQUIPMENT: Kettlebell

PRIME MOVERS: Biceps, deltoids, quadriceps

ASSISTANT MOVERS: Gluteal muscles, hamstrings, triceps

STABILIZERS: Core muscles, rotator cuff muscles, forearm muscles

PREREQUISITE EXERCISES: Dumbbell biceps curl (page 41), barbell squat (page 70), shoulder press (page 35)

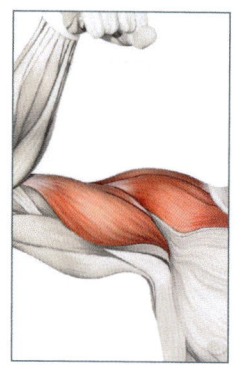

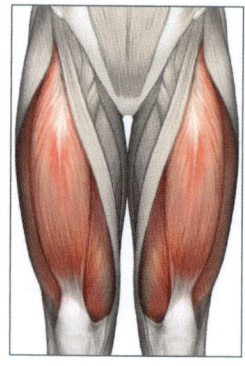

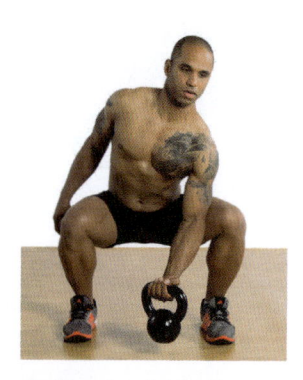

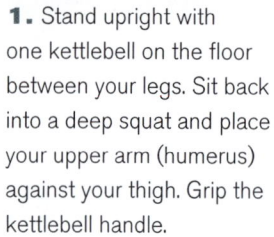

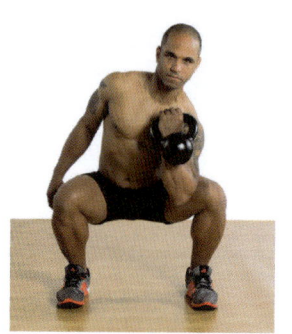

1. Stand upright with one kettlebell on the floor between your legs. Sit back into a deep squat and place your upper arm (humerus) against your thigh. Grip the kettlebell handle.

2–4. Flex your elbow and curl the kettlebell, then extend your legs to stand. Press the kettlebell up until your arm is fully extended.

Reverse all of the steps until you're in a deep squat with the kettlebell on the floor.

FULL-BODY MOVEMENTS 107

Kettlebell Sit-Up & Stand

EQUIPMENT: Kettlebell
PRIME MOVERS: Rectus abdominis, internal and external obliques, quadriceps
ASSIST MOVERS: Gluteal muscles, pectoral muscles, latissimus dorsi
STABILIZERS: Calves, biceps, triceps, core muscles, forearm muscles
PREREQUISITE EXERCISES: Sit-up (page 52), barbell squat (page 70)

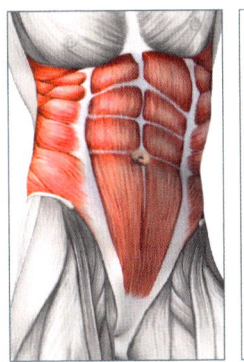

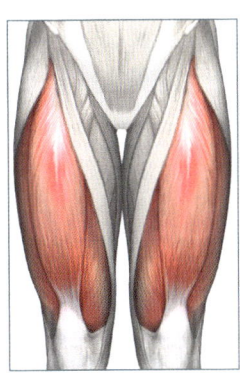

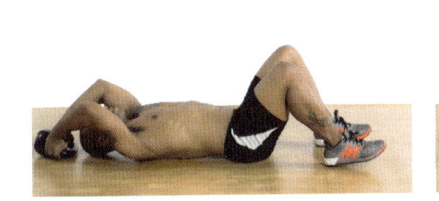

1. Lie face-up with your knees bent and your feet on the floor. Hold one kettlebell in both hands with your arms behind your head.

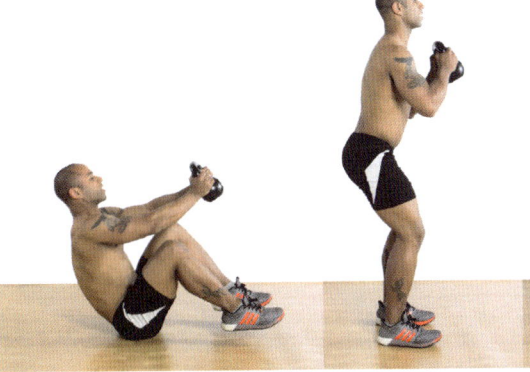

2. Swing your arms forward and use the momentum of the arm swing to assist in sitting up. As you approach the top of the sit-up, continue to use the momentum of the arm swing to assist in standing up.

Squat back down and then lower back into the starting position.

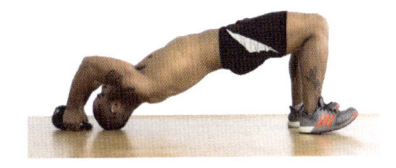

PROGRESSION

- Add a neck bridge to the beginning of the movement.

REGRESSION

- Stop when you reach the sit-up; don't stand up.

NOTES

- This movement relies on momentum and quickly transitioning from one segment to the next.

Burpee

EQUIPMENT: None
PRIME MOVERS: Pectoralis major, quadriceps
ASSISTANT MOVERS: Triceps, gluteal muscles, calves
STABILIZERS: Core muscles, rotator cuff muscles, biceps, triceps
PREREQUISITE EXERCISES: Barbell squat (page 70), push-up (page 13)

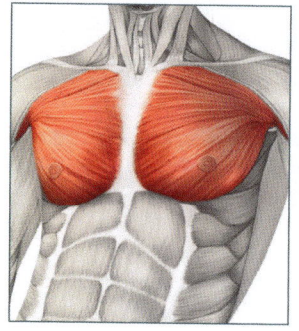

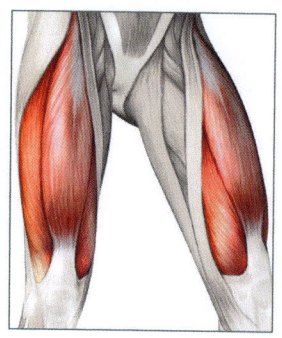

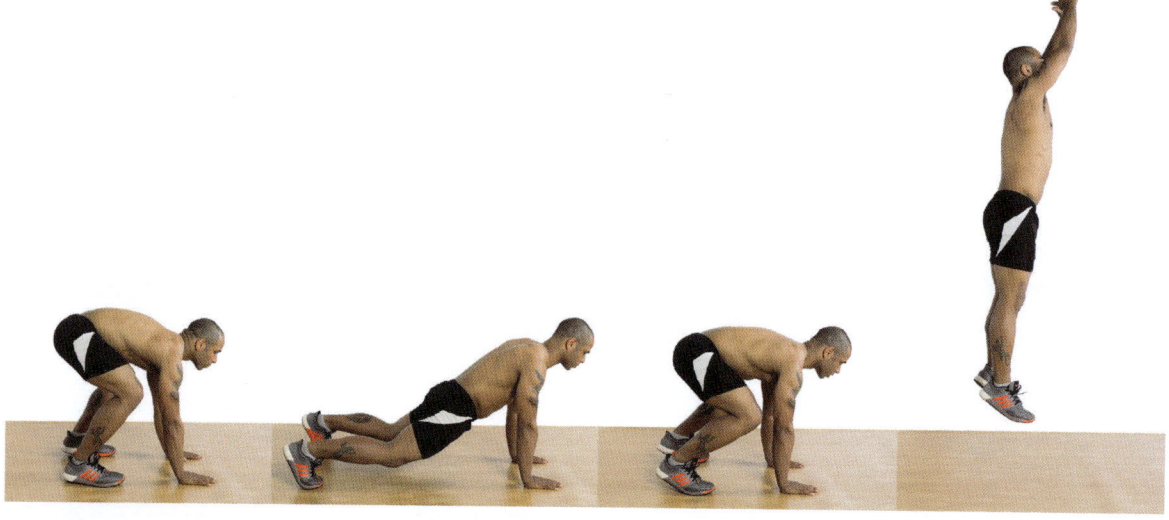

1–2. Stand upright. Squat and place your hands on the floor.

3. As your hands hit the floor, shoot both legs out behind you at the same time, using your arms to keep you stable. You should wind up at the top of a push-up position.

4. Pull both legs in at the same time.

5. Straighten your legs into a jump.

PROGRESSION

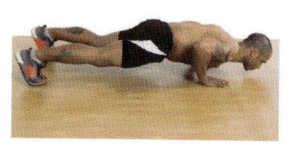

- Add a push-up at the bottom.

Sandbag Squat & Throw

EQUIPMENT: Sandbag

PRIME MOVERS: Quadriceps, pectoralis major

ASSISTANT MOVERS: Anterior deltoids, triceps, gluteal muscles

STABILIZERS: Core muscles

PREREQUISITE EXERCISE: Barbell squat (page 70)

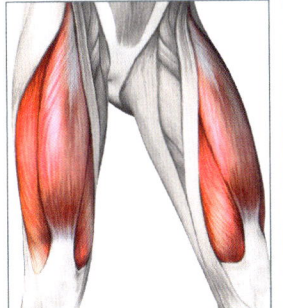

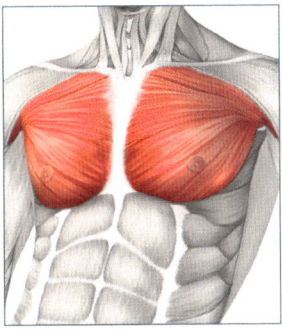

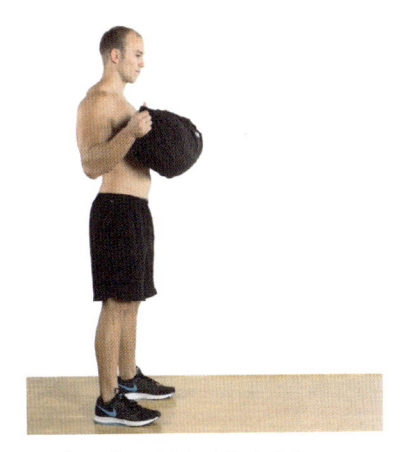

FULL-BODY MOVEMENTS 109

1. Stand upright while holding a sandbag at chest height.

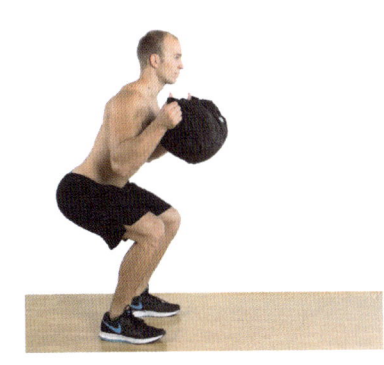

2. Sit back into a full squat.

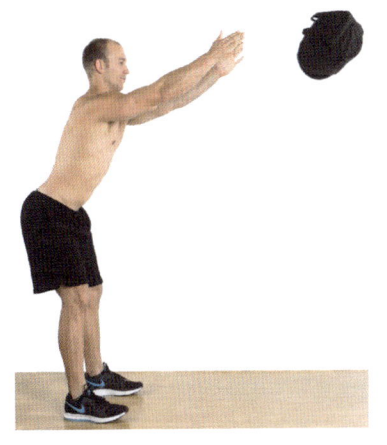

3. Powerfully pushing through your heels and extending up from the squat, use the momentum to powerfully press the sandbag forward and throw it as far as you can.

NOTES

- You can try to throw the sandbag with a wide or minimal arc.

Explosive Medicine Ball Full-Body Throw

EQUIPMENT: Medicine ball

PRIME MOVERS: Quadriceps, pectoralis major

ASSISTANT MOVERS: Gluteal muscles, triceps, anterior deltoids, calves

STABILIZERS: Core muscles

PREREQUISITE EXERCISES: Barbell squat (page 70), explosive squat jump (page 73), bench press (page 14)

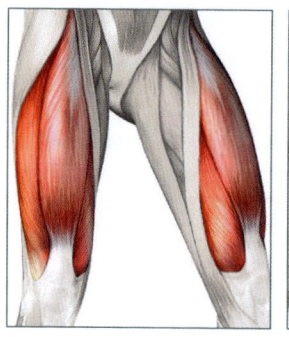

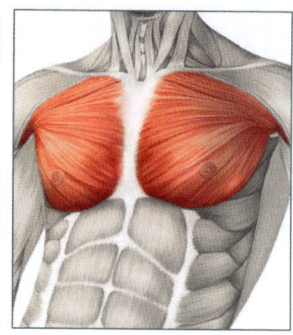

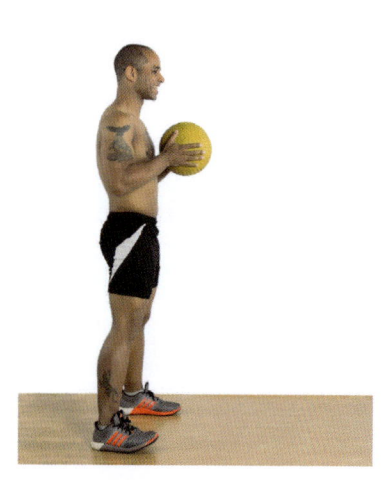

1. Stand upright and hold a medicine ball at chest height.

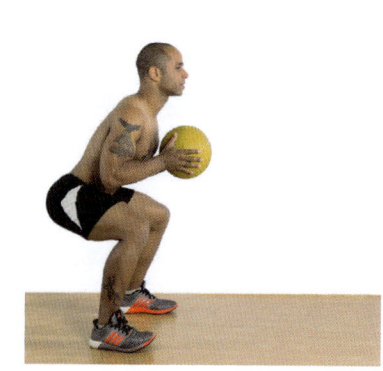

2. Lower into a full squat.

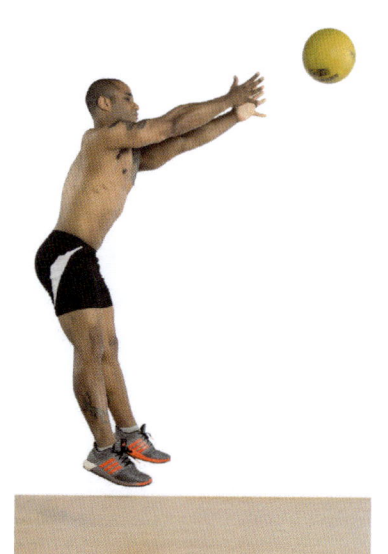

3. Explode up into a jump and powerfully extend both arms forward, throwing the ball as far as you can.

NOTES
- It's important to perform each repetition as quickly and powerfully as you can.

FULL-BODY MOVEMENTS 111

Explosive High Pull

EQUIPMENT: Barbell
PRIME MOVERS: Deltoids, trapezius, quadriceps
ASSISTANT MOVERS: Gluteal muscles, calves, biceps
STABILIZERS: Core muscles, forearm muscles
PREREQUISITE EXERCISE: Upright row (page 36)

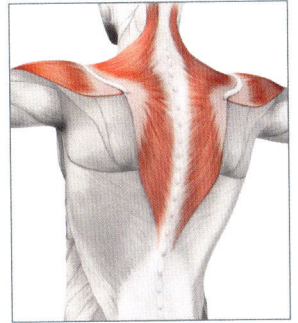

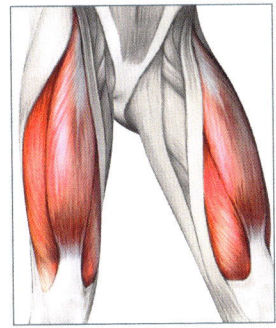

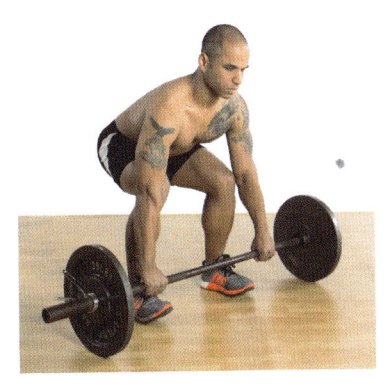

1. Stand behind a bar that's resting either on the floor or an elevated surface. Your feet should be hip- to shoulder-width apart with your toes pointing straight ahead. Sit back and grip the bar with your palms facing you.

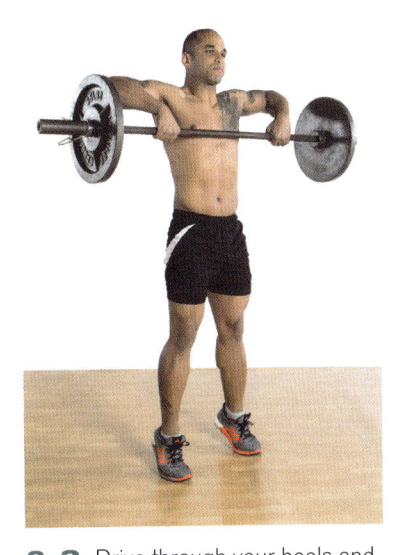

2–3. Drive through your heels and powerfully extend your legs and torso. As you approach an upright posture, use the momentum to pull the barbell up to chest height. As your legs reach full extension and the bar approaches chest height, plantarflex your ankles. You may also drive your hips forward slightly but make sure to maintain a neutral spine.

Lower the weight all the way back.

NOTES

- It's important to perform each repetition as quickly and powerfully as you can.

FREEWEIGHT TRAINING ANATOMY

Explosive Kettlebell Clean

EQUIPMENT: Kettlebell

PRIME MOVERS: Deltoids, trapezius

ASSISTANT MOVERS: Erector spinae, biceps, gluteal muscles

STABILIZERS: Core muscles

PREREQUISITE EXERCISE: Kettlebell swing (page 103)

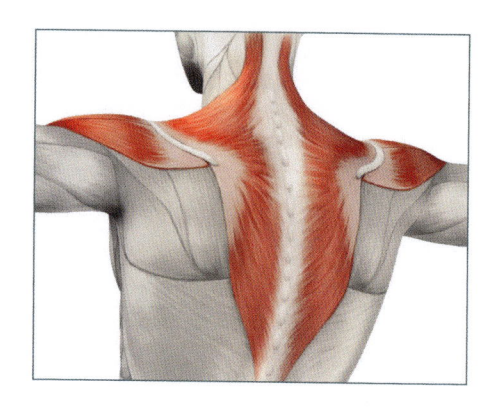

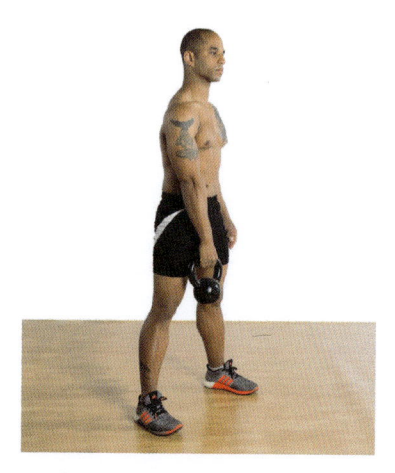

PROGRESSION

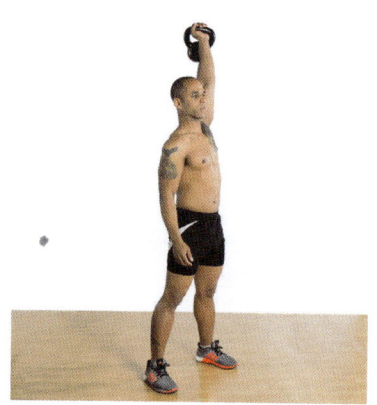

- Add a press to the movement.

1. Stand upright holding one kettlebell in one hand.

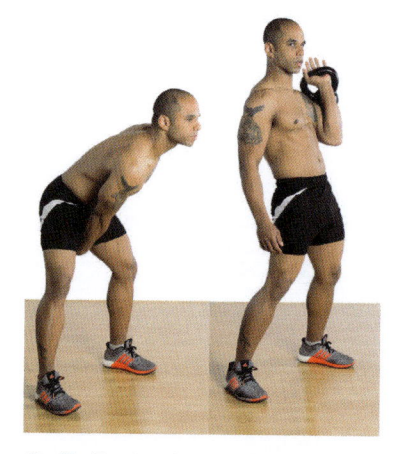

2–3. Begin a kettlebell swing. As your arm approaches being parallel to the floor, shoot your hips forward, bend your knees slightly, and pull the kettlebell back, turning your elbow in and flicking the kettle back. At the top of the movement, your arm should be resting on your trunk and your palm should be in a neutral position while holding the kettlebell.

NOTES

- It's important to perform each repetition as quickly and powerfully as you can.

FULL-BODY MOVEMENTS 113

Explosive Single-Arm Dumbbell Snatch

EQUIPMENT: Dumbbell

PRIME MOVERS: Deltoids, quadriceps

ASSISTANT MOVERS: Biceps, calves, gluteal muscles

STABILIZERS: Core muscles, rotator cuff muscles, forearm muscles

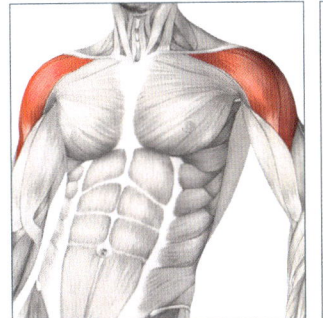

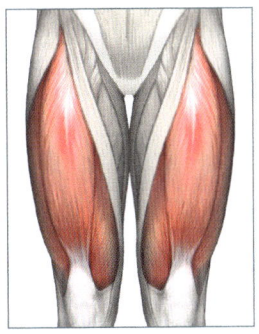

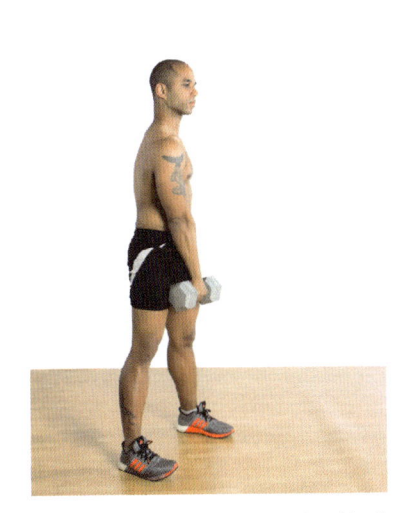

1. Stand upright holding a dumbbell in one hand with the arm fully extended and hanging between your legs.

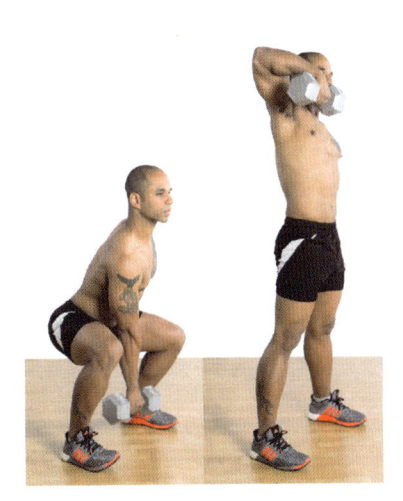

2–3. Sit back into a squat with the dumbbell remaining in place at your midline. At the bottom of the movement, you should be in a three-quarter squat. Driving through your heels, extend your legs and use the momentum generated from your leg extension to pull the dumbbell up by abducting your upper arm. The dumbbell should be close to your trunk the entire time.

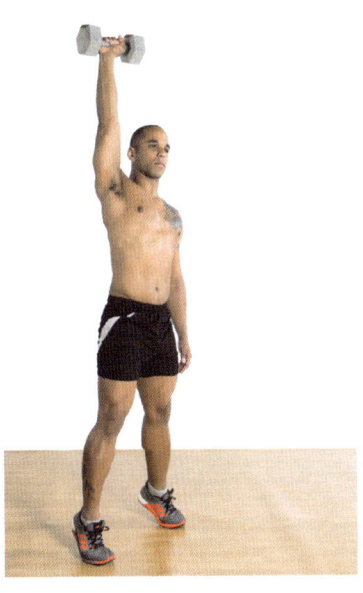

4. As the dumbbell reaches chest height, continue to use the momentum generated to fully extend your arm up toward the ceiling. Lower your arm back to the starting position.

NOTES
- It's important to perform each repetition as quickly and powerfully as you can.

Explosive Kettlebell Snatch

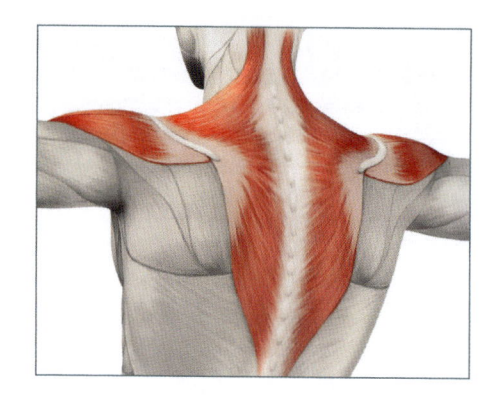

EQUIPMENT: Kettlebell

PRIME MOVERS: Deltoids, trapezius

ASSISTANT MOVERS: Erector spinae, biceps, gluteal muscles

STABILIZERS: Core muscles, forearm muscles

PREREQUISITE EXERCISE: Kettlebell swing (page 103)

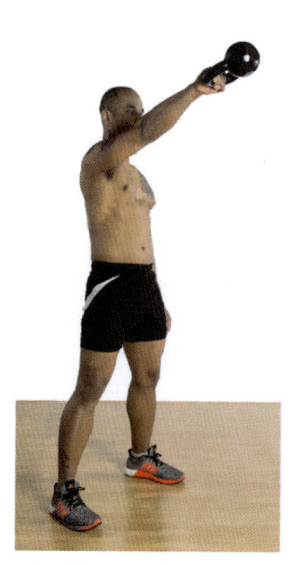

REGRESSION

- Perform the same steps while holding a dumbbell.

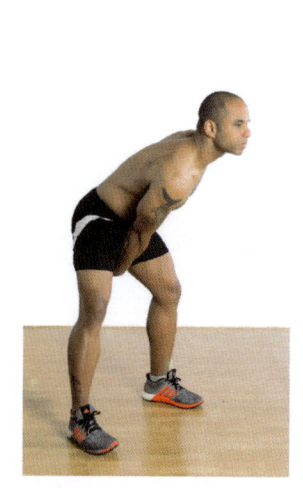

1–3. Stand upright holding one kettlebell in one hand. Begin a kettlebell swing. As you approach the top of the swing, pull the kettlebell back by horizontally abducting your arm. As your arm approaches your chest, powerfully extend your arm straight up.

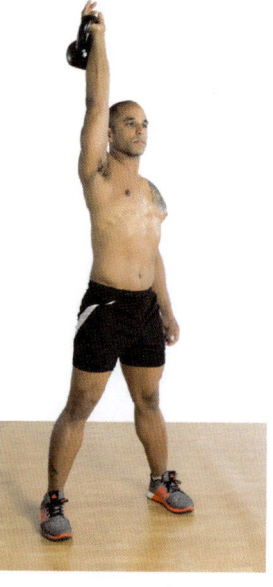

Lower back into a swing.

NOTES

- It's important to perform each repetition as quickly and powerfully as you can.

PART 3
THE PROGRAMS

GETTING STARTED

While the majority of this book is focused on resistance training, there are a few other essential components to your exercise program. Warm-up, cardio, and cool-down are all important to include in your exercise programming. Warm-ups and cool-downs are necessary in order avoid injuries. Cardio is also important to help strengthen your heart and maintain your weight.

Warming Up

It's extremely important to warm up your body before engaging in any kind of exercise. Not only does doing so get your body ready for the activity at hand, it also plays a big role in preventing injury.

There are three basic ways to warm up. A *general warm-up* can be any movement (such as jogging in place, jumping rope, or jumping jacks) that increases the heart rate and overall blood flow throughout the body. Fitness equipment, such as elliptical machines, bikes, and treadmills, are also excellent. General warm-ups are especially effective prior to cardiovascular activities. Warm-ups should last 5 to 10 minutes and your heart rate should reach between 90 to 110 beats per minute (bpm). If your heart rate falls below 90, increase the intensity of your warm-up; if it exceeds 110, decrease the intensity.

Movement preparation is a method of stimulating the nervous system by targeting individual joints. This allows you to "wake up" your muscles and prepare your body for exercise. The focus of movement preparation is to mobilize the joints that rely on mobility and stabilize the joints that rely on stability. Movement preparation is a good way to warm up if you have any joint injuries or muscle imbalances. It's also good as preparation for functional and athletic movements.

Dynamic stretching is a movement-based method of stretching designed to take joints through their normal range of motion while still increasing body temperature and heart rate. Unlike static stretches, dynamic stretches aren't held. This is a good way to warm up if you're preparing for movements and activities that require a large range of motion. It also helps to loosen tight or stiff muscles prior to exercise.

Time permitting, you can benefit greatly from a combination of these three types of warm-ups. Doing so will thoroughly prepare your body for exercise. If you combine the three, begin with a 5-minute general warm-up, followed by the movement preparation and then dynamic stretching.

MOVEMENT PREPARATION

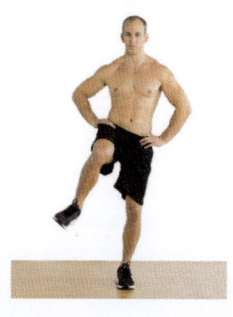

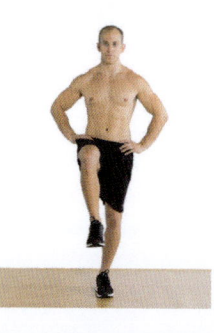

Foot Circle

This improves ankle mobility.

1–2. Do 10 to 15 complete circles in a clockwise direction and then 10 to 15 complete circles in a counterclockwise direction.

3. Alternate dorsiflexion (flexing your foot) and plantarflexion (pointing your foot) 10 to 15 times.

Side Lunge

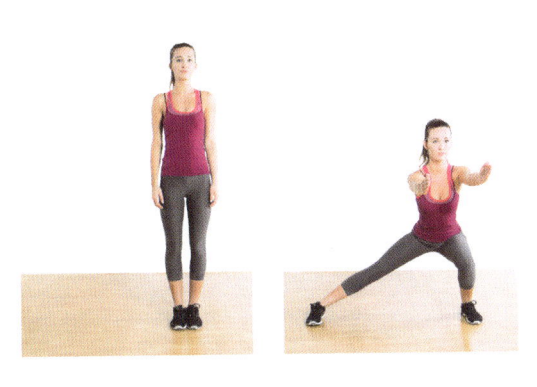

This works on knee stability.

1. Stand upright with both feet together.

2. Step to your right side, bend your right knee, sit back, and extend your arms forward. The other leg should be completely straight.

Repeat to the other side.

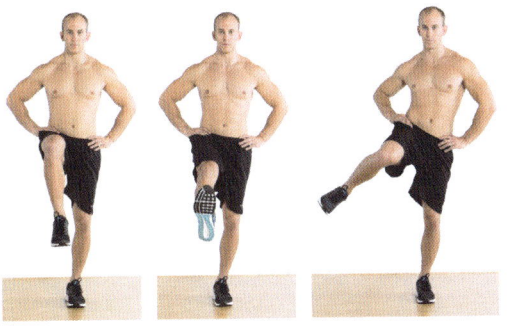

Hip Mobility

1. While standing, raise your right knee to hip height, keeping your thigh parallel to the floor. Maintain this position for the duration of the exercise.

2. Fully straighten your knee and then bend it.

3. Internally rotate your hip and then externally rotate it.

4. Move your knee across your body and then take it out to the side.

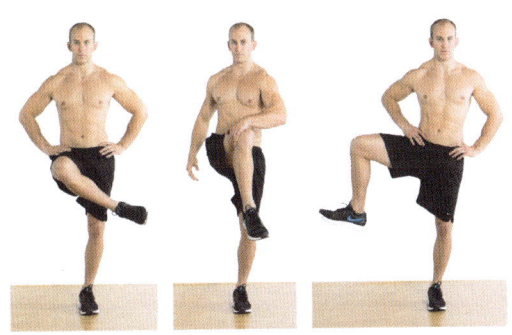

Plank

This focuses on trunk stability. See page 60 for instructions on how to perform this exercise.

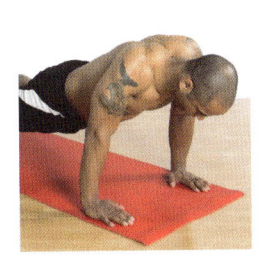

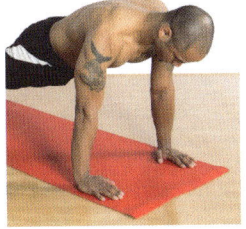

Scapular Push-Up

1. From a push-up position, retract (pinch) your shoulder blades together. Make sure to keep your arms straight.

2. Protract (release) your shoulders back to the starting position.

DYNAMIC STRETCHES

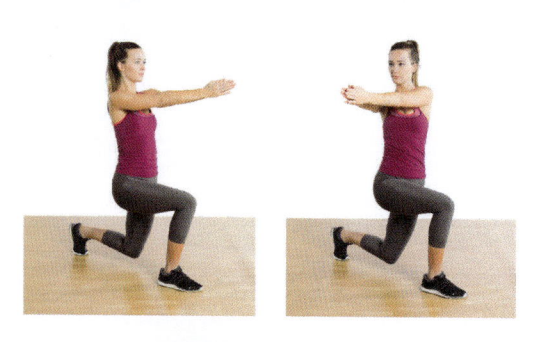

Lunge Rotate

1. From standing, step your right foot forward into a lunge.
2. Now rotate to your right side.

Repeat to the other side.

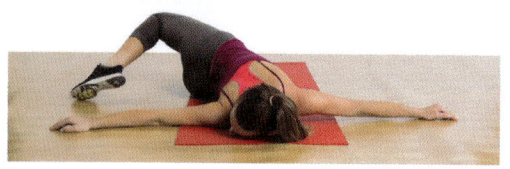

Prone Leg Rotation

1. Lie facedown on the floor with your arms out to the side.
2. Bend your right knee and rotate your torso to the left until your foot touches the floor.

Repeat with the other side.

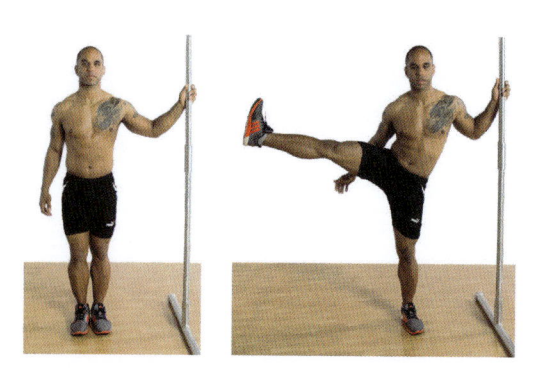

Leg Swing Side

1. Stand next to a wall, chair, or other object for support.

2–3. Swing your leg across your body as much as you comfortably can, and then swing your leg back out the side.

Repeat, then switch sides.

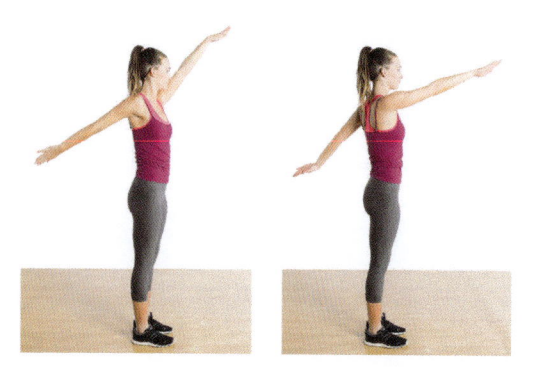

Arm Swing

1. From standing, extend one arm fully overhead and the other arm fully back behind you.
2. Switch positions then continue alternating.

Cardio

In addition to resistance training, cardiovascular activity such as running, rowing, jumping rope, and cycling plays a major role in increasing one's fitness level. Cardiovascular activity is any activity that uses oxygen as the body's primary source of energy. This is achieved by continuously performing submaximal movements over an extended period of time.

Cardiovascular work is characterized by repetitive work at a low to moderate intensity with little to no rest. It generally has two primary functions. The first is to strengthen the heart. As our hearts get stronger, our ability to extract oxygen from our blood (VO2 max) increases. The second function is weight loss. Cardiovascular work can be designed to be sustained for as little as 10 minutes to longer than one hour. Your cardio can be completed in short and very intense intervals, or longer but moderate-intensity sessions. The higher the intensity, the less time is required.

| RPE SCALE ||
RATING	PERCEIVED EXERTION
10	Maximum Effort
9	Very high Intensity
7–8	High Intensity
4–6	Moderate Intensity
2–3	Low Intensity
1	Minimum Intensity

It's important to be aware of your heart rate and/or rate of perceived exertion (RPE) when engaging in cardiovascular work. The level of intensity is inversely proportional to the amount of time you should spend. This means that if you exercise at a higher intensity, you'll require less time than exercising at a lower intensity.

Stretching & Cooling Down

Stretching can kill two birds with one stone as it gives you the opportunity to cool down while also incorporating your flexibility training. All stretches should be held for 15 to 30 seconds. Move the joint to the point where you feel mild discomfort; you shouldn't be in pain. If a muscle is particularly tight, you can hold the stretch for 30 seconds, release, and stretch again for another 30 seconds.

TARGET HEART RATE (THR)

Your THR is the heart rate goal that you set up for cardiovascular activity. To begin, you'll have to determine your maximum heart rate (HRMax), which is the highest that your heart rate should get with exercise.

>   HRMax = 220 − age

For example, a 32-year-old would have a maximum heart rate of 188.

Once you have your maximum heart rate, you must then determine your intensity level.

>   60% THR = HRMax x .6
>
>   70% THR = HRMax x .7
>
>   80% THR = HRMax x .8

The percentage of your HRMax is directly related to the RPE scale above.

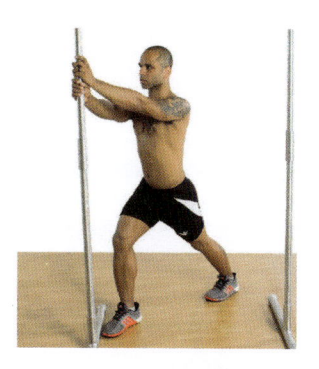

Calf Stretch (Gastrocnemius)

The Position: Facing a wall, place your hands on the wall with your arms fully extended. Split your legs so that one leg is in front and the other is extended behind you. Bend your lead leg until you feel the stretch in the rear calf. The rear heel should be on the floor with the toes pointed straight ahead; the knee should be fully extended the entire time.

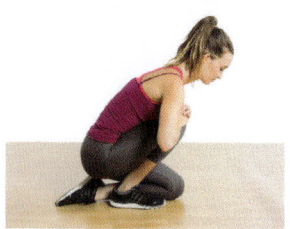

Calf Stretch (Soleus)

The Position: Stand with one foot in front of the other and sit back on the heel of your rear leg. Pull the lead foot back until you feel a stretch in your calves. Make sure that the heel of your lead leg is touching the floor the entire time. To intensify the stretch, pull the lead foot back more. To make the stretch less intense, move the foot forward. Switch sides.

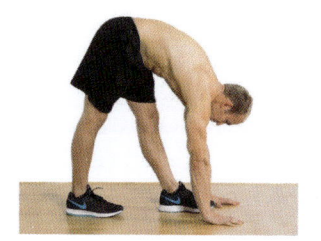

Hamstrings Stretch

The Position: Stand with one foot in front of the other. Bend both knees and place both hands on the floor. Keeping your hands on the floor, straighten both legs to stretch the lead leg.

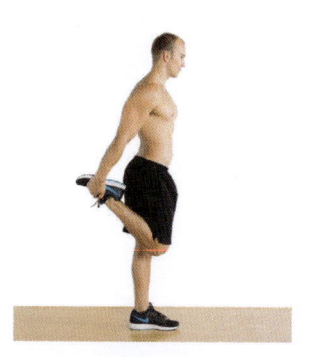

Quads Stretch

The Position: Standing upright, bend one knee and grip your foot with the same-side hand. Pull the heel toward you with your knee pointing straight down.

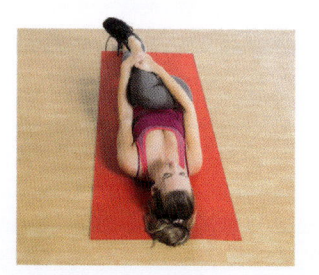

Glutes Stretch

The Position: Lie on your back with both legs straight. Without rotating your torso, pull one knee up and across toward the opposite shoulder. Switch sides.

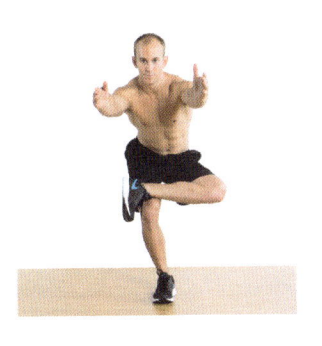

Glutes/Piriformis Stretch 1

The Position: Stand with your feet together and place your left ankle on your right thigh, just above your knee. Extend your arms forward, parallel to the floor, and sit back as much as you comfortably can. Hold. Switch sides.

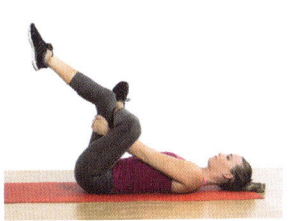

Glutes/Piriformis Stretch 2

The Position: Lie on your back with both knees bent. Place your left ankle on your right thigh. With both hands, grab your right thigh and pull in. Switch sides.

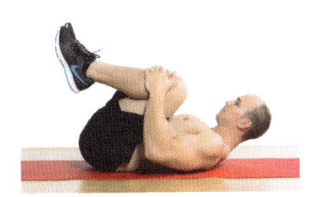

Lower Back Stretch

The Position: Lie on your back and pull both knees into your chest.

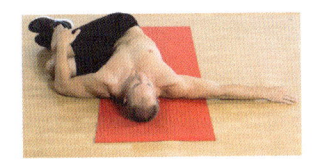

Obliques Stretch

The Position: Lie on your back and lift both legs so that your hips and knees are both bent 90 degrees. Lower your knees and hips to one side until your legs touch the floor. Place your hand on the top leg and gently pull down. Extend your other arm so that both shoulders are flat on the floor. Switch sides.

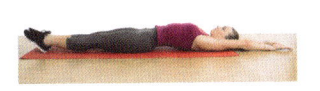

Abdominal Stretch 1

The Position: Lie on your back with your arms and legs extended. Reach your arms back toward the wall behind you while simultaneously pointing your toes forward to the wall in front of you.

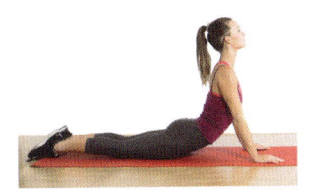

Abdominal Stretch 2

The Position: Lie facedown and place your palms on the floor next to you. Press your palms into the floor, lifting your trunk off the floor.

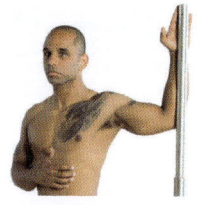

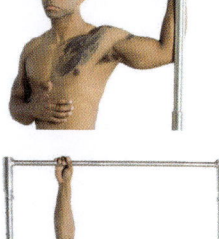

Pec Stretch

1. Stand next to a wall with your arm bent 90 degrees and your upper arm parallel to the floor. Place your forearm against the wall.

2. Rotate in the opposite direction while maintaining contact with the wall.

Lats Stretch

The Position: Stand underneath a doorframe pull-up bar and grip the bar with one hand. Keeping your arm straight, shoot your hips out to one side. Then shoot them out to the other side.

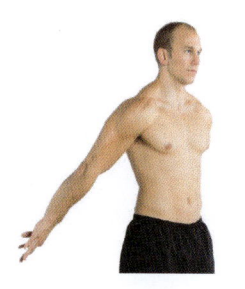

Biceps Stretch

The Position: Stand upright with both arms at your sides and thumbs facing forward. Internally rotate your thumbs and extend your elbows as much as you can. Keeping both the rotation and the extension, reach your arms as far backward as you can.

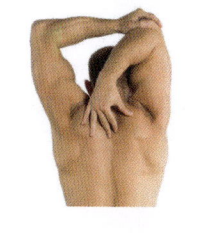

Triceps Stretch

The Position: Extend your right arm overhead and then bend your elbow to touch the base of your neck. Use your other arm to gently push down on the elbow to intensify the stretch. Switch sides.

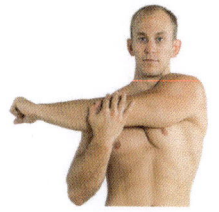

Deltoids Stretch

The Position: Take one arm across your chest, using your other arm to grab behind your elbow and gently pull your arm in to intensify the stretch. Switch sides.

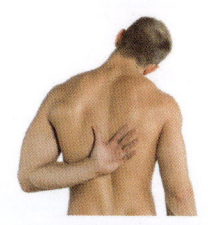

Traps Stretch

The Position: Bend your left arm and place it behind your back. Tilt your right ear to your right shoulder. Switch sides.

PROGRAMMING FOR YOUR GOALS

In addition to understanding the exercises and their muscles and function, it's important to understand how to properly utilize them in an exercise program. There are a number of variables to consider when designing an exercise program. The variables can change dramatically depending on the goal, so the first step in designing an exercise program is to determine your fitness goals. Once you determine these goals, you can apply the specific variables and implement the most effective fitness program for your goals.

Variables

Load: This is the amount of weight, usually represented in pounds (lbs) or kilograms (kg). An easy way to determine the correct load is to relate it to the number of repetitions required. If an exercise calls for 8 repetitions, for example, the load should be such that you can complete 8 repetitions with good form. It should be heavy enough that you cannot complete 9 to 10 repetitions with good form. If you can, then you should increase the weight and try again.

Repetitions (Reps): One repetition is represented as an exercise performed from the starting position to its midpoint and back to its starting position. Repetitions as an exercise variable is represented as the number of consecutive repetitions performed without rest.

Sets: One set consists of a group of repetitions.

Volume: The volume of an exercise or workout is the load multiplied by the sets multiplied by the repetitions. This represents the total amount of work completed in an exercise or workout.

Tempo: Tempo refers to the speed of the movement. Tempo will usually consist of 3 numbers referring to the number of seconds to perform the concentric, isometric, and eccentric actions. As an example, if we're performing a pull-up, a tempo of 1-1-3 would mean that the pulling-up portion should be completed in 1 second, the isometric hold at the top of the movement should be held for 1 second, and the lowering portion should be completed over 3 seconds.

Rest: This refers to the amount of rest between sets of an exercise.

Number of exercises: This refers to the total number of different exercises to include in each exercise session.

Sessions/week: This refers to the total number of workouts per week.

Body parts/week: This refers to the number of times per week that you should focus on each body part.

Types of movements: This refers to which movements to stress.

Cardio: This refers to the type and intensity of cardio for the goal.

Goals

Determining your goal is key to customizing the right exercise program for you. Below is a chart of seven common goals and how you can easily put together a program that works for you.

	GENERAL FITNESS	ULTIMATE STRENGTH	EXPLOSIVE POWER	MASS BUILDING	ATHLETE	WEIGHT LOSS	SHREDDING
Load	Moderate	Heavy; increase the load over time	Moderate but on the heavy side	Moderate to heavy	Moderate to heavy	Moderate	Moderate to high
Reps per exercise	8-12	3-6	3-6	6-12	10-15	10-12	8-10
Sets per exercise	4-5	4-5	4-5	5-6	3-5	4-5	3-4
Volume	Medium to high	Low to medium	Low to medium	High	Moderate	Medium to high	High
Tempo	2-1-3	2-2-4	1-1-1	2-2-3	1-1-2	1-1-3	2-2-3
Rest	2-5 minutes	2-5 minutes	2-5 minutes	1-3 minutes	1-4 minutes	Short to 2 minutes	1-3 minutes
Number of exercises	8-10	4-6	6-8	8-12	8	8-10	8-12
Sessions/week	3-5	4-5	1-2	5-6	4-6	4-5	4-6
Body parts/week	1-2	1-2	1-2	2	1-2	1-2	2

General fitness: When focusing on general fitness, you can be very flexible in the types of movements. A combination of movements and modalities is ideal, but a majority of the exercises should be multi-joint; full-body movements are recommended. Consistency is the key when putting together a general fitness program.

Strength: Multi-joint exercises like squats, deadlifts, and bench presses are best for developing strength. Full-body movements are also great for developing overall strength. Isolation exercises can help but should be used as secondary exercises. Lifting heavy weight and increasing your numbers over time are the keys to developing strength. Allow a minimum of 2–3 days of recovery time before working the same body parts. You can work on more than one muscle group within a workout, but begin with the larger, multi-joint movements before working on the smaller, single-joint movements.

Explosive power: Choose explosive movements that use multiple joints. The key is performing these exercises with maximum power. This means that you must perform each repetition in the shortest time possible. There's a higher risk of injury with these exercises so proper form is essential. While these movements are meant to be explosive, you must still be in control of your body.

Mass building: Movements to build mass should be a combination of single- and multi-joint exercises. Volume and intensity are keys to building mass. Additionally, it's important to continually increase the loads week to week.

Athlete: Choose a combination of power, full-body, core, and multi-joint movements. While every sport has different specific requirements, power and functional strength are important for almost every sport.

Weight loss: Any weight-loss program should be accompanied by cardiovascular exercise and a clean diet.

Shredding: Pick a combination of single- and multi-joint movements. This is a very high-intensity program and should be accompanied by cardiovascular exercise and a clean diet.

Training Programs

There are a number of ways to design and implement a fitness program. Below are the most common, as well as a description of how to best utilize them.

SINGLE SET

With single sets, you perform all of the required sets for each exercise before moving on to the next exercise. You should rest completely in between each set.

Good for: General fitness, strength building.

SUPERSETS

Supersets combine 2 exercises that are performed back to back with little to no rest. Sets are performed in pairs. Supersets can be designed to work opposing muscle groups (biceps/triceps), upper body and lower body, or the same muscle group.

Good for: Weight loss, shredding, athletes.

CIRCUIT TRAINING

Circuit training consists of performing a series of exercises consecutively with little or no rest in between exercises. A circuit can consist of 3 to 10 different exercises. Try to cover the entire body with a mix of upper-body, lower-body, and core movements.

Good for: Weight loss, shredding, athletes.

DROP SETS

Drop sets involve performing 2 to 3 consecutive sets of an exercise with little to no rest. Take a 35-pound shoulder press as an example: You'd begin with 10 repetitions with the 35 pounds. After the first set, you'd drop the weight to 25 or 30 pounds and perform another 8 to 10 repetitions. After the second set, you may drop even further and perform another 8 to 10 repetitions.

Good for: Mass building, shredding.

TABATA

Tabata has a very specific protocol. Each exercise consists of eight 20-second rounds broken up with 10-second rest periods. During the working periods, you should move as quickly as you can. The objective of tabata is to maximize your intensity and use the short rest periods to recover enough to begin again. You should find a speed that works for you, so if anything is too difficult, slow down; if it's easy, speed it up.

Good for: Shredding, weight loss, athletes.

EXERCISE PROGRAMS

If you're going to use the programs in this section, there are a few things to keep in mind. First is determining your initial load. Since everyone is different, you'll have to determine this number on your own. The initial load should be whatever weight is appropriate in order to perform the number of repetitions. As the program progresses, you should try to increase the load by 5 to 10 pounds every one to two weeks. If the increase is heavier than you can manage, you may lower the weight.

If you're lifting heavy weights, it's best to perform 1 to 3 sets with lighter weights in order to warm up for the movement and to develop greater neuromuscular control. It's also important to be mindful of the tempo and rest periods. These are both important and will lead to different training effects depending on how they're utilized.

If you aren't comfortable with a particular exercise or you don't have access to a specific piece of equipment, simply replace it with an exercise from the same category.

General Fitness Program

	EXERCISE	WEEK 1	WEEK 2	WEEK 3	WEEK 4	WEEK 5	WEEK 6
		\multicolumn{6}{c}{Sets x Reps/Duration}
DAY 1	**Bench Press** tempo: 2-2-3 | rest: 2 min	3x10	3x10	3x10	3x10	3x10	3x10
	Dumbbell Press tempo: 2-2-3 | rest: 90 sec	3x10	3x10	3x10	3x10	3x10	3x10
	Decline Dumbbell Pullover tempo: 2-2-3 | rest: 90 sec	3x12	3x12	3x12	3x12	3x12	3x12
	Barbell Row tempo: 1-2-3 | rest: 90 sec	3x12	3x12	3x12	3x12	3x12	3x12
	One-Arm Dumbbell Row tempo: 1-2-3 | rest: 90 sec	3x10	3x10	3x10	3x10	3x10	3x10
	Straight-Arm Dumbbell Extension tempo: 2-2-3 | rest: 60 sec	3x10	3x10	3x10	3x10	3x10	3x10
	Physioball Crunch tempo: 1-1-2 | rest: 30 sec	3x30	3x30	3x30	3x30	3x30	3x30
	Plank tempo: 1-30-1 | rest: 60 sec	3x1	3x1	3x1	3x1	3x1	3x1

EXERCISE PROGRAMS

	EXERCISE	WEEK 1	WEEK 2	WEEK 3	WEEK 4	WEEK 5	WEEK 6
		Sets x Reps/Duration					
DAY 2	**Dumbbell Biceps Curl** Tempo: 1-2-3 | Rest: 60 sec	3x12	3x12	3x12	3x12	3x12	3x12
	Dumbbell Hammer Curl tempo: 1-2-3 | rest: 60 sec	3x12	3x12	3x12	3x12	3x12	3x12
	Barbell Biceps Curl tempo: 2-2-3 | rest: 60 sec	3x10	3x10	3x10	3x10	3x10	3x10
	Dumbbell Kickback tempo: 2-2-3 | rest: 60 sec	3x12	3x12	3x12	3x12	3x12	3x12
	Kettlebell Triceps Extension tempo: 2-2-3 | rest: 60 sec	3x12	3x12	3x12	3x12	3x12	3x12
	Bent-Over T Extension tempo: 1-1-3 | rest: 60 sec	3x10	3x10	3x10	3x10	3x10	3x10
	Sit-Up tempo: 1-1-3 | rest: 60 sec	3x10	3x10	3x10	3x10	3x10	3x10
	Total-Body Crunch tempo: 1-1-3 | rest: 60 sec	3x15	3x15	3x15	3x15	3x15	3x15
DAY 3	**Shoulder Press** tempo: 1-2-3 | rest: 60 sec	3x12	3x12	3x12	3x12	3x12	3x12
	Dumbbell Lateral Raise tempo: 1-1-3 | rest: 60 sec	3x10	3x10	3x10	3x10	3x10	3x10
	Dumbbell Reverse Fly tempo: 1-1-2 | rest: 60 sec	3x12	3x12	3x12	3x12	3x12	3x12
	Barbell Squat tempo: 2-2-3 | rest: 60 sec	3x10	3x10	3x10	3x10	3x10	3x10
	Dumbbell Lunge tempo: 2-2-3 | rest: 60 sec	3x8	3x8	3x8	3x8	3x8	3x8
	Dumbbell Front Raise tempo: 1-2-3 | rest: 60 sec	3x12	3x12	3x12	3x12	3x12	3x12
	Superman tempo: 1-2-3 | rest: 30 sec	3x12	3x12	3x12	3x12	3x12	3x12
	Single-Leg Bridge tempo: 1-2-3 | rest: 30 sec	3x12	3x12	3x12	3x12	3x12	3x12

Ultimate Strength

	EXERCISE	WEEK 1	WEEK 2	WEEK 3	WEEK 4	WEEK 5	WEEK 6
		Sets x Reps					
DAY 1	**Deadlift** tempo: 2-2-3 | rest: 2–4 min	4x8	4x7	4x6	4x6	4x5	4x5
	Barbell Squat tempo: 2-2-3 | rest: 2–4 min	4x8	4x8	4x7	4x7	4x6	4x6
	Dumbbell Lunge tempo: 1-2-2 | rest: 90 sec	4x8	4x8	4x8	4x7	4x7	4x7
	Straight-Leg Deadlift tempo: 2-2-3 | rest: 90 sec	4x8	4x8	4x7	4x7	4x7	4x7
DAY 2	**Bench Press** tempo: 2-2-3 | rest: 2–4 min	4x8	4x8	4x7	4x7	4x7	4x7
	Barbell Row tempo: 1-2-3 | rest: 2–4 min	4x8	4x8	4x6	4x6	4x6	4x6
	Dumbbell Press tempo: 2-2-3 | rest: 2–4 min	4x8	4x8	4x6	4x6	4x6	4x6
	One-Arm Dumbbell Row tempo: 2-2-3 | rest: 2–4 min	4x8	4x8	4x6	4x6	4x6	4x6
	Decline Dumbbell Pullover tempo: 2-2-3 | rest: 60–90 sec	4x8	4x8	4x6	4x6	4x6	4x6
DAY 3	**Shoulder Press** tempo: 2-2-3 | rest: 2–4 min	4x8	4x8	4x6	4x6	4x6	4x6
	Barbell Biceps Curl tempo: 2-2-3 | rest: 2–4 min	4x8	4x7	4x7	4x6	4x6	4x5
	Dumbbell Biceps Curl tempo: 2-2-3 | rest: 2 min	4x8	4x7	4x7	4x6	4x6	4x5
	Close Grip Bench Press tempo: 2-2-3 | rest: 2 min	4x8	4x8	4x6	4x6	4x6	4x6
	Dumbbell Lateral Raise tempo: 2-2-3 | rest: 90 sec	4x8	4x8	4x6	4x6	4x6	4x6
	Explosive High Pull tempo: 2-2-3 | rest: 2–4 min	4x8	4x8	4x6	4x6	4x6	4x6
DAY 3	Repeat Day 1						
DAY 4	Repeat Day 2						

Explosive Power

	EXERCISE	WEEK 1	WEEK 2	WEEK 3	WEEK 4	WEEK 5	WEEK 6
		Sets X Reps					
DAY 1	**Explosive Push-Up** tempo: fast | rest: 90 sec	4x10	4x10	4x15	4x15	4x15	4x20
	Explosive Squat Jump tempo: fast | rest: 90 sec	4x15	4x15	4x20	4x20	4x20	4x20
	Kettlebell Swing tempo: fast | rest: 90 sec	4x12	4x12	4x12	4x12	4x15	4x15
	Sandbag Squat and Throw tempo: fast | rest: 1–2 min	3x8	3x8	3x10	3x10	3x12	3x12
	Kettlebell Sit-Up & Stand tempo: fast | rest: 90 sec	3x8	3x8	3x10	3x10	3x12	3x12
	Burpee tempo: fast | rest: 1 min	4x12	4x12	4x15	4x15	4x20	4x20
DAY 2	**Explosive Kettlebell Clean** tempo: fast | rest: 1 min	4x8	4x8	4x8	4x8	4x8	4x8
	Explosive Push Press tempo: fast | rest: 1 min	4x8	4x8	4x8	4x8	4x8	4x8
	Explosive Kettlebell Snatch tempo: fast | rest: 1–2 min	4x8	4x8	4x7	4x6	4x6	4x6
	Explosive High Pull tempo: fast | rest: 1–2 min	4x8	4x8	4x7	4x6	4x6	4x6
	Explosive Medicine Ball Full-Body Throw tempo: fast | rest: 1–2 min	4x8	4x8	4x8	4x8	4x8	4x8
DAY 3	**Repeat Day 1**						
DAY 4	**Repeat Day 2**						

Mass Builder

	EXERCISE	WEEK 1	WEEK 2	WEEK 3	WEEK 4	WEEK 5	WEEK 6
		\multicolumn{6}{c}{Sets x Reps}					
DAY 1	**Bench Press** tempo: 2-2-3 | rest: 90 sec	4x10	4x10	4x10	4x10	4x10	4x10
	Dumbbell Press tempo: 2-2-3 | rest: 90 sec	4x12	4x12	4x10	4x10	4x10	4x10
	Dumbbell Reverse Fly tempo: 2-2-3 | rest 90 sec	4x12	4x12	4x10	4x10	4x10	4x10
	Close-Grip Bench Press tempo: 2-2-3 | rest: 90 sec	4x10	4x10	4x10	4x8	4x8	4x8
	Kettlebell Triceps Extension tempo: 2-2-3 | rest: 60 sec	4x10	4x10	4x10	4x10	4x10	4x10
	Kettlebell Press tempo: 2-2-3 | rest: 60 sec	4x10	4x10	4x10	4x10	4x10	4x10
	Dumbbell Kickback tempo: 1-1-3 | rest: 60 sec	4x12	4x12	4x10	4x10	4x10	4x10
DAY 2	**Barbell Row** tempo: 1-2-3 | rest: 90 sec	4x10	4x10	4x8	4x8	4x8	4x8
	One-Arm Dumbbell Row tempo: 2-2-3 | rest: 90 sec	4x12	4x10	4x10	4x10	4x10	4x10
	Decline Dumbbell Pullover tempo: 3-2-3 | rest: 90 sec	4x10	4x10	4x10	4x10	4x10	4x10
	Barbell Biceps Curl tempo: 2-2-3 | rest: 90 sec	4x12	4x12	4x10	4x10	4x10	4x10
	Dumbbell Biceps Curl tempo: 2-2-3 | rest: 60–90 sec	4x12	4x12	4x10	4x10	4x10	4x10
	Pull-Up tempo: 2-1-3 | rest: 90 sec	4x10	4x10	4x10	4x10	4x10	4x10
	Dumbbell Hammer Curl tempo: 1-2-3 | rest: 60 sec	4x12	4x12	4x10	4x10	4x10	4x10

EXERCISE PROGRAMS

	EXERCISE	WEEK 1	WEEK 2	WEEK 3	WEEK 4	WEEK 5	WEEK 6
		\multicolumn{6}{c}{Sets x Reps}
DAY 3	**Dumbbell Squat** tempo: 2-2-3 | rest: 90 seconds	4x10	4x10	4x10	4x8	4x8	4x8
	Deadlift tempo: 2-2-3 | rest: 90 sec	4x10	4x10	4x10	4x8	4x8	4x8
	Dumbbell Lunge tempo: 1-2-3 | rest: 60 sec	4x10	4x10	4x10	4x10	4x10	4x10
	Shoulder Press tempo: 2-2-3 | rest: 60–90 sec	4x12	4x12	4x10	4x10	4x10	4x10
	Dumbbell Lateral Raise tempo: 1-2-3 | rest: 60 sec	4x12	4x12	4x10	4x10	4x10	4x10
	Upright Row tempo: 2-2-3 | rest: 60 sec	4x12	4x10	4x10	4x10	4x10	4x10
	Straight-Leg Deadlift tempo: 2-2-3 | rest: 60 sec	4x10	4x10	4x10	4x10	4x10	4x10
	Dumbbell Front Raise tempo: 2-2-3 | rest: 60 sec	4x10	4x10	4x10	4x10	4x10	4x10
DAY 4	**Repeat Day 1**						
DAY 5	**Repeat Day 2**						
DAY 6	**Repeat Day 3**						

Shredding

Supersets involve performing a pair of exercises back to back. Try to limit the rest time between each pair of exercises.

EXERCISE	WEEK 1	WEEK 2	WEEK 3	WEEK 4	WEEK 5	WEEK 6
	\multicolumn{6}{c}{Sets x Reps}
1a. Dumbbell Press 15 tempo: 1-1-2 | rest: 0	3x12	3x12	3x10	3x8	3x8	3x8
1b. Dumbbell Fly 16 tempo: 1-1-2 | rest: 20 sec	3x10	3x10	3x10	3x10	3x10	3x10
2a. Barbell Row 31 tempo: 1-2-3 | rest: 0	3x12	3x12	3x12	3x10	3x10	3x10
2b. One-Arm Dumbbell Row 23 tempo: 1-2-2 | rest: 20 sec	3x12	3x12	3x12	3x10	3x10	3x10
3a. Bench Press 14 tempo: 1-1-2 | rest: 0	3x12	3x12	3x12	3x10	3x10	3x10
3b. Two-Arm Dumbbell Row 24 tempo: 1-1-2 | rest: 20 sec	3x15	3x15	3x12	3x12	3x12	3x12
4a. Dumbbell Squat 70 tempo: 1-1-2 | rest: 0	3x12	3x12	3x12	3x12	3x12	3x12
4b. Dumbbell Lunge 71 tempo: 1-2-2 | rest: 20 sec	3x10	3x10	3x10	3x10	3x10	3x10
5a. Kettlebell Swing 103 rest: 0	3x15	3x15	3x15	3x15	3x15	3x15
5b. Plank 60 tempo: 1-30-1 | rest: 20 sec	3x1	3x1	3x1	3x1	3x1	3x1
6a. Kettlebell Renegade Row 102 rest: 0	3x10	3x10	3x10	3x10	3x10	3x10
6b. Total-Body Crunch 54 tempo: 1-1-2 | rest: 20 sec	3x15	3x15	3x15	3x15	3x15	3x15

DAY 1

- 15 second rest between each pair of exercises
- Perform 3 sets of each exercise.

EXERCISE PROGRAMS

	EXERCISE	WEEK 1	WEEK 2	WEEK 3	WEEK 4	WEEK 5	WEEK 6
		\multicolumn{6}{c|}{Sets x Reps}					
DAY 2	1a. Dumbbell Biceps Curl 41 tempo: 1-1-2 | rest: 0	3x12	3x12	3x12	3x10	3x10	3x10
	1b. Dumbbell Hammer Curl 42 tempo: 1-1-2 | rest: 20 sec	3x10	3x10	3x10	3x10	3x10	3x10
	2a. Close-Grip Bench Press 48 tempo: 1-1-2 | rest 0	3x10	3x10	3x10	3x10	3x10	3x10
	2b. Dumbbell Kickback 49 46 tempo: 1-1-2 | rest: 20 sec	3x12	3x12	3x12	3x12	3x12	3x12
	3a. Upright Row 36 tempo: 1-1-2 | rest: 0	3x10	3x10	3x10	3x10	3x10	3x10
	3b. Dumbbell Lateral Raise 33 tempo: 1-1-2 | rest: 20 sec	3x8	3x8	3x8	3x8	3x8	3x8
	4a. Barbell Biceps Curl 41 tempo: 1-2-2 | rest: 0	3x12	3x12	3x12	3x10	3x10	3x10
	4b. Kettlebell Triceps Extension 49 tempo: 1-1-2 | rest: 20 sec	3x10	3x10	3x10	3x10	3x10	3x10
	5a. Dumbbell Front Raise 34 tempo: 1-1-2 | rest: 0	3x10	3x10	3x10	3x10	3x10	3x10
	5b. Dumbbell Reverse Fly 38 tempo: 1-1-2 | rest: 20 sec	3x10	3x10	3x10	3x10	3x10	3x10
	6a. Explosive Kettlebell Clean 112 tempo: fast | rest: 0	3x10	3x10	3x10	3x10	3x10	3x10
	6b. Explosive Squat Jump 73 tempo: fast | rest: 20 sec	3x15	3x15	3x15	3x15	3x15	3x15
DAY 3	**Repeat Day 1**						
DAY 4	**Repeat Day 2**						

Athlete's Workout

	EXERCISE	WEEK 1	WEEK 2	WEEK 3	WEEK 4	WEEK 5	WEEK 6
		Sets x Reps					
DAY 1	**Deadlift** tempo: 1-2-3 | rest: 90 sec	3x10	3x10	3x8	3x8	3x8	3x8
	Barbell Squat tempo: 1-1-3 | rest: 90 sec	3x10	3x10	3x10	3x10	3x10	3x10
	Kettlebell Swing rest: 60–90 sec	3x15	3x15	3x15	3x15	3x15	3x15
	Kettlebell Renegade Row rest: 60–90 sec	3x8	3x8	3x8	3x8	3x8	3x8
	Turkish Get-Up rest: 2 min	2x5	2x5	3x5	3x8	3x8	3x8
	Straight-Leg Deadlift tempo: 2-1-3 | rest: 90 sec	3x10	3x10	3x10	3x10	3x10	3x10
	Dumbbell Press tempo: 1-1-2 | rest: 60–90 sec	3x10	3x10	3x10	3x10	3x10	3x10
	Plank tempo: 1-30-1 | rest: 60 sec	3x1	3x1	3x1	3x1	3x1	3x1
DAY 2	**Explosive Push-Up** tempo: fast | rest: 60–90 sec	3x10	3x10	3x10	3x10	3x10	3x10
	Explosive Squat Jump tempo: fast | rest: 60–90 sec	3x15	3x15	3x20	3x20	3x20	3x20
	Explosive Push Press tempo: fast | rest: 60–90 sec	3x12	3x12	3x12	3x12	3x12	3x12
	Explosive Kettlebell Snatch tempo: fast | rest: 60–90 sec	3x6	3x6	3x8	3x8	3x8	3x8
	Explosive Kettlebell Clean tempo: fast | rest: 60–90 sec	3x10	3x10	3x10	3x10	3x10	3x10
	Burpee tempo: fast | rest: 60–90 sec	3x20	3x20	3x20	3x20	3x20	3x20
	Kettlebell Sit-Up & Stand tempo: fast | rest: 90 sec	3x8	3x8	3x8	3x8	3x8	3x8
	Plank tempo: 1-60-1 | rest: 60 sec	2x1	2x1	3x1	3x1	3x1	3x1
DAY 3	Repeat Day 1						
DAY 4	Repeat Day 2						

Weight Loss

Circuit training involves performing a series of exercises consecutively with little rest in between. The number of rounds represents the number of times that you should complete the circuit.

	EXERCISE	WEEK 1	WEEK 2	WEEK 3	WEEK 4	WEEK 5	WEEK 6
		\multicolumn{6}{c}{Reps}
DAY 1	Burpee	10	10	15	15	20	20
	Two-Arm Dumbbell Row	12	12	12	10	10	10
	Push-Up	15	15	15	15	15	15
	Dumbbell Biceps Curl	12	12	12	12	12	12
	Dumbbell Lateral Raise	10	10	10	10	10	10
	Burpee	10	10	15	15	20	20
	Dumbbell Press	12	12	10	10	10	10
	Forward Lunge	10	10	10	10	10	10
	Total-Body Crunch	15	15	15	15	15	15
	Kettlebell Triceps Extension	12	12	12	12	12	12
	ROUNDS	2	2	3	3	4	4
DAY 2	Explosive Squat Jump	15	15	15	15	15	15
	Bench Dip	15	15	15	15	15	15
	Kettlebell Swing	15	15	15	15	15	15
	Kneeling Rollout	12	12	12	12	12	12
	Explosive High Pull	12	12	12	12	12	12
	Explosive Squat Jump	15	15	15	15	15	15
	Turkish Get-Up	8	8	8	8	8	8
	Squat Curl & Press	10	10	10	10	10	10
	Explosive Push Press	12	12	12	12	12	12
	Straight-Leg Deadlift	12	12	12	12	12	12
	ROUNDS	2	2	3	3	4	4
DAY 3	Repeat Day 1						
DAY 4	Repeat Day 2						

INDEX

Abdominal (stomach) muscles, 50; exercises, 52–67; stretches, 121

Abdominal Stretch 1 & 2, 121

Abduction, 3

Adduction, 3

Adductor (leg) muscles, 94; exercises, 95–96

Antagonist muscles, 5

Arm muscles. *See* Biceps muscles; Forearm muscles; Triceps muscles

Arm Swing, 118

Assistant movers, 5, 8

Athlete's workout, as goal, 124; program, 134

Back muscles. *See* Latissimus dorsi muscles; Lower back muscles; Upper back muscles

Barbell Row, 31

Barbell Squat, 70

Barbells, 9

Bench Dip, 45

Bench Press, 14

Bench Pullover, 17

Bent-Over T Extension, 47

Biceps (arm) muscles, 40; exercises, 41–43; stretches, 122

Biceps Stretch, 122

Bodyweight, 9

Breathing, 5

Bridges, 84

Burpee, 108

Butt muscles. *See* Gluteal muscles

Calf muscles, 78; exercises 79–80; stretches, 120

Calf Stretch (Gastrocnemius), 120

Calf Stretch (Soleus), 120

Cardio, 119

Catch position, 10

Chest muscles. *See* Pectoral muscles

Circuit training, 125

Cleans, 112

Close-Grip Bench Press, 48

Compound exercises, 4

Concentric contraction, 4

Consistency principle, 6

Contraction, of muscle, 4

Cooling down, 119

Core (trunk) muscles, 51; exercises, 52–67; stretches, 121

Crossover Crunch, 53

Crunches, 53, 54, 57

Curls: arm, 41, 42, 43, 98; leg, 75, 77; wrist, 86

Deadlift (basic), 101

Deadlifts, 76, 101

Decline Dumbbell Pullover, 25

Deltoid (shoulder) muscles, 32; exercises, 33–39; stretches, 122

Deltoids Stretch, 122

Dips, 45

Dorsiflexion & Foot Circle, 93

Drop sets, 125

Dumbbell Biceps Curl, 41

Dumbbell Fly, 16

Dumbbell Front Raise, 34

Dumbbell Hammer Curl, 42

Dumbbell Kickback, 46

Dumbbell Lateral Raise, 33

Dumbbell Leg Lift, 67

Dumbbell Lunge, 71
Dumbbell Press, 15
Dumbbell Reverse Fly, 38
Dumbbell Scapular Retraction, 30
Dumbbell Shrug, 29
Dumbbells, 9
Dynamic stretching, 116; exercises, 118

Eccentric contraction, 4
Efficiency principle, 6
Equipment, 8–9
Eversion, 4
Exercises, 12–114; positions, 9–10; programs, 126–35; stretching/cooling down, 119–22; types, 4; warming up, 116–18
Explosive High Pull, 111
Explosive Kettlebell Clean, 112
Explosive Kettlebell Snatch, 114
Explosive Medicine Ball Full-Body Throw, 110
Explosive power, as goal, 124; program, 129
Explosive Push Press, 39
Explosive Push-Up, 20
Explosive Single-Arm Dumbbell Snatch, 113
Explosive Squat Jump, 73
Extension, of muscle, 3
External Rotation & Press, 90
External Rotation to Shoulder Press, 91

Fitness overview, 3–7; concepts, 6–7; principles, 5–6
Flexion, of muscle, 3
Floor Leg Extension, 69
Flys, 16, 38
Foot Circle, 116
Forearm muscles, 85; exercises, 86–88
Freeweight training equipment, 89
Full-body movements, 97; exercises, 98–114
Functional exercises, 4

General fitness: as goal, 124; program, 126–27
General warm-ups, 116
Gluteal (butt) muscles, 81; exercises, 82–84; stretches, 120
Glutes Stretch, 120
Glutes/Piriformis Stretch 1 & 2, 121
Goals, fitness, 124

Hamstring (leg) muscles, 74; exercises, 75–77; stretches, 120
Hamstrings Stretch, 120
Hip flexor muscles, 51; exercises, 52–67
Hip Mobility, 117
Hyperextension, 3
Hypertrophy, 3

Inversion, 4
Isolation exercises, 4
Isometric contraction, 4

Kettlebell Anyhow, 106
Kettlebell Kneeling Concentration Curl, 43
Kettlebell Lunge Passthrough, 72
Kettlebell Press, 18
Kettlebell Renegade Row, 102
Kettlebell Sit-Up, 58
Kettlebell Sit-Up & Stand, 107
Kettlebell Swing, 103
Kettlebell Triceps Extension, 49
Kettlebells, 9
Kneeling Rollout, 63

Latissimus dorsi (back) muscles, 21; exercises, 22–27; stretches, 122
Lats Stretch, 122
Leg Lowering, 65

Leg muscles. *See* Adductor muscles; Calf muscles; Hamstring muscles; Hip flexor muscles; Quadriceps muscles; Shin muscles

Leg Raise, 66

Leg Swing Side, 118

Load, 123

Lower back muscles, 50; exercises, 52–67; stretches, 121

Lower Back Stretch, 121

Lunge Rotate, 118

Lunges, 71, 72, 95, 99, 100, 117, 118

Mass building, as goal, 124; program, 130–31

Maximum heart rate (HR max), 119

Medicine Ball Seated Rotation, 55

Medicine Ball Wraparound, 56

Medicine balls, 9

Movement: components, 5; exercises, 116–17; positions, 9–10; preparation, 116; types, 3–4

Muscle contraction, 4

Muscle extension, 3

Muscle flexion, 3

Muscles, overview, 2. *See also specific muscles*

Nordic Hamstring Curl, 77

Obliques Stretch, 121

One-Arm Dumbbell Row, 23

Overtraining, 7

Pec Stretch, 122

Pectoral (chest) muscles, 12; exercises, 13–20; stretches, 122

Periodization, 6–7

Physioball Crunch, 57

Physioball Hamstring Curl, 75

Physioball Plank with Arm Extension, 62

Physioball Push-Up, 19

Physioballs, 9

Planks (basic), 60, 117

Planks, 60, 61, 62, 96, 117

Plateaus in exercise program, 6

Plyometrics, 7

Positions, 9–10

Presses: barbells, 39, 91; bench, 14, 48; dumbbells, 15, 35, 98; external rotation, 90; kettlebells, 18

Prime movers, 5, 8

Program, exercise, 126–35

Progression principle, 6

Pronation/Supination, 88

Prone Leg Rotation, 118

Prone position, 10

Pullovers, 17, 25

Pull-Up (basic), 27

Push-Up (basic), 13

Push-ups, 13, 19, 20, 117

Quadriceps (leg) muscles, 68; 69–73; stretches, 120

Quadruped Kickback, 82

Quadruped position, 10

Quads Stretch, 120

Raises, 33, 34, 66, 79, 80

Range of motion (ROM), 4

Rate of perceived exertion (RPE), 119

Rear Deltoid Dumbbell Row, 37

Repetitions (reps), 123

Resistance training, 3

Rest, 123

Rest/recovery principle, 6

Rotation, 4

Rotator cuff muscles, 89; exercises, 90–91

Rows: barbells, 31, 36; dumbbells, 23, 24, 37; kettlebells, 26, 102

INDEX

Sandbag Lunge & Rotation, 100
Sandbag Squat & Throw, 109
Sandbags, 9
Scapular Push-Up, 117
Seated Calf Raise, 80
Seated Kettlebell Toss, 64
Seated position, 9
Sets, 123
Shin muscles, 92; exercises, 93
Shoulder muscles. *See* Deltoid muscles; Rotator cuff muscles
Shoulder Press, 35
Shredding, as goal, 124; program, 132–33
Side Lunge with Sword Draw, 99
Side Lunge, 95, 117
Side lying positions, 10
Side Plank, 61
Side Plank with Elevated Bottom Leg, 96
Side-Lying Abduction, 83
Single-Leg Bridge, 84
Single-Leg Kettlebell Row, 26
Single sets, 125
Sit-Up (basic), 52
Sit-ups, 52, 58, 107
Snatches, 113, 114
Specificity principle, 6
Squat, Curl & Press, 98
Squats, 70, 73, 98, 109
Stabilizer muscles, 5, 8
Standing positions, 9
Stomach muscles. *See* Abdominal muscles
Straight-Arm Dumbbell Extension, 22
Straight-Leg Deadlift, 76
Strength, as goal, 124; program, 128
Stretches, 120–22
Superman, 59

Supersets, 125
Supine position, 10

Tabatas, 125
Target heart rate (THR), 119
Tempo, 123
Throws, 109, 110
Toe Raise, 79
Total-Body Crunch, 54
Training programs, 125
Traps Stretch, 122
Triceps (arm) muscles, 44; exercises, 45–49; stretches, 122
Triceps Stretch, 122
Trunk muscles. *See* Abdominal muscles; Core muscles; Hip flexor muscles; Lower back muscles
Turkish Get-Up, 104–105
Two-Arm Dumbbell Row, 24

Upper back muscles, 28; exercises, 29–31
Upright Row, 36

Variables, in program design, 123
Volume, 123

Warming up, 116–18
Weight loss, as goal, 124; program, 135
Wrist Curl, 86
Wrist Extension, 87

ACKNOWLEDGMENTS

First, I'd like to thank Ana, Nicholas, and Crystal for providing such a strong support system. I couldn't ask for a better family and I'm incredibly lucky to have you in my life. I'd like to thank my parents, Eddie and Donna, for being so loving and hard-working.

I'd also like to thank Ajarn Coban, Sandra, and everyone at Team Coban for giving me such a great opportunity and providing a home away from home.

In my time in the fitness industry, I've met so many wonderful people, and so many people have been instrumental in my success. A special thank-you to everyone whom I've met along this journey—it has been an awesome one for me.

Finally, I want to thank everyone at Ulysses Press for their support and confidence in me. It's a tremendous honor and I'm thankful for the opportunity.

ABOUT THE AUTHOR

Ryan George has been involved in the fitness industry since 2001. He has worked with a diverse client base that includes everyone from celebrities to students, children to geriatric clients, and professional athletes to post-rehab patients. Ryan has specialized certifications in integrated flexibility, sports conditioning, kettlebells, and TRX. Ryan also works as an instructor for the World Instructor Training Schools (WITS), helping to educate and develop future generations of trainers. Ryan has made a number of media appearances, including those on ABC and CBS News as a fitness expert.

Ryan has been practicing Muay Thai since 2007 and is an amateur Muay Thai fighter and trainer under the legendary fighter/trainer Coban Lookchaomaesaithong. To date, he has a record of 4-1.

The author of *Doorframe Pull-Up Bar Workouts* (Ulysses Press, 2014), Ryan currently cohosts *The GymWits*, a weekly fitness podcast that can be found on iTunes or at www.TheGymWits.com. More information about Ryan can be found at www.RyanGeorgeFitness.com.

Printed in Great Britain
by Amazon